STP 1090

Continuous Anesthesia Gas Monitoring

John Hedley-Whyte and Peter W. Thompson

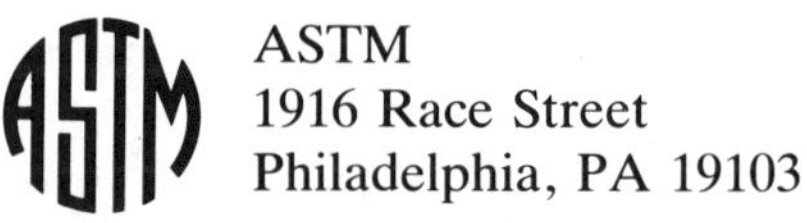

ASTM
1916 Race Street
Philadelphia, PA 19103

Library of Congress Cataloging-in-Publication Data

Continuous anesthesia gas monitoring/[edited by] John Hedley-Whyte
and Peter W. Thompson.
(STP; 1090)
Papers presented at the symposium held in London on Feb. 21,
1989.
Includes bibliographical references.
ISBN 0-8031-1394-3
1. Anesthesia—Congresses.   2. Transcutaneous blood gas
monitoring—Congresses.   I. Hedley-Whyte, John.   II. Thompson,
Peter W.   III. Series: ASTM special technical publication; 1090.
RD82.C67   1990
617.9′6—dc20   90-337
                                                                     CIP

NOTE

The Society is not responsible, as a body,
for the statements and opinions
advanced in this publication.

Peer Review Policy

Each paper published in this volume was evaluated by three peer reviewers. The authors addressed all of the reviewers' comments to the satisfaction of both the technical editor(s) and the ASTM Committee on Publications.

The quality of the papers in this publication reflects not only the obvious efforts of the authors and the technical editor(s), but also the work of these peer reviewers. The ASTM Committee on Publications acknowledges with appreciation their dedication and contribution of time and effort on behalf of ASTM.

Printed in Ann Arbor, MI
May 1990

Foreword

This publication, *Continuous Anesthesia Gas Monitoring,* contains papers presented at the symposium of the same name held in London, England, on 21 February 1989. The symposium was sponsored by ASTM Committee F-29 on Anesthetic and Respiratory Equipment and ISO Committee TC-121 on Anaesthetic and Respiratory Equipment. Dr. John Hedley-Whyte, West Roxbury V.A. Medical Center, Boston, MA, and Dr. Peter W. Thompson, University Hospital of Wales, Heath Park, Cardiff, Wales, United Kingdom, presided as symposium cochairmen and were editors of this publication.

Contents

John Hedley-Whyte[1]

Overview: Technology Assessment in Medicine and Surgery and the Voluntary Consensus Standards Writing Process

International standards activity in anesthesia and intensive care commenced in Technical Committee 121 on Anaesthetic and Respiratory Equipment of the International Organization for Standardization (ISO) in 1966 and was initially dependent on prior work by national standards writing bodies, especially those in the United Kingdom (British Standards Institution, or BSI), United States (American National Standards Institute, or ANSI) and France (Association Française de Normalisation, or AFNOR). National work has continued, but the United States committee was transferred to the American Society for Testing and Materials (ASTM) in 1983 [1].

More recently, many of the ISO standards have been written jointly by delegates from the 20 participating countries and 24 observer countries with the corresponding Committee 62D on Electromedical Equipment of the International Electrotechnical Commission (IEC), reflecting the increasing role of electronics in medical equipment. At present there are 26 published international standards under the purview of TC 121 and 10 draft international standards which are also purchasable [2].

Anesthetic mishaps frequently result in anoxic brain damage or death. The outcome of anoxic brain-damaged patients is strikingly inferior to the outcome of patients with prolonged coma after craniocerebral trauma [3]. In a recent review of 1,175 anesthetic-related closed malpractice claims in the United States, reviewers were asked if the poor outcomes would have been preventable by proper use of additional monitoring devices. In over 1000 patient records, sufficient information was available to judge whether or not the mortality or morbidity was preventable by the use of additional monitoring devices, and in almost a third of patients (31.5%) it would have been. The costs of legal judgment or settlement of mishaps judged preventable by additional monitoring were eleven times costlier ($p < 0.01$) than those after mishaps not so preventable. Pulse oximetry plus capnometry were deemed to be most useful in mishap prevention, and together these two technologies were considered potentially able to prevent 93% of the preventable mishaps [4]. Continuous anesthesia vapor monitoring techniques were among other monitors deemed valuable in the remaining cases.

Medical equipment technologies evolve through three stages—development, diffusion, and established practice. ASTM Committee F-29 on Anesthetic and Respiratory Equipment and ISO Technical Committee 121 felt that continuous anesthesia vapor monitoring at the end of the 1980s was in the process of diffusion, and that experts should opine on whether a transition to the third stage was merited. Hence this volume.

If continuous anesthesia vapor monitoring becomes established practice, it would be wise to heed the advice of Dr. Henry Krakauer of the United States Health Care Financing Administration to the Technology Assessment Group of the Harvard University School of

[1]Departments of Anaesthesia and Health Policy and Management, Harvard University, Boston, MA 02132.

Public Health: "As it [technology] undergoes refinement and as new competing technologies enter into practice, information must continue to accrue to permit the continuing comparison of the relative merits of alternative procedures, and the adjustment of incentives to assure the most effective utilization of resources" [5]. For these resources are indeed limited [6].

Acknowledgments

The editorial staff and publications committee of ASTM have been invaluable in the preparation of this publication. The continued help of Professor Frederick Mosteller, Director, Technology Assessment Group, Department of Health Policy and Management, Harvard University School of Public Health and Roger I. Lee Professor of Mathematical Statistics, Emeritus, and Professor Robert J. Blendon, Chairman of the Department of Health Policy and Management, Harvard University School of Public Health, is gratefully acknowledged.

References

[1] Hedley-Whyte, J., *Clinical Anaesthesiology*, Vol. 2, No. 2, 1988, pp. 379–389.
[2] Stratton, R. R., "Report of the Secretariat on Progress of Work Since the 17th Meeting Held in Helsinki in July 1988," ISO TC 121 Doc. No. N 476, British Standards Institution (BSI), 2 Park Street, London, W1A 2 BS, 22 August 1989.
[3] Groswasser, Z., Cohen, M., and Costeff, H., *Archives of Physical Medicine and Rehabilitation*, Vol. 70, 1989, pp. 186–188.
[4] Tinker, J. H., Dull, D. L., Caplan, R. A., Ward, R. J., and Cheney, F. W., *Anesthesiology*, Vol. 71, 1989, pp. 541–546.
[5] Krakauer, H., "An Approach to the Systematic Assessment of Medical Technologies," report to the Registries and Datasets Subgroup, Technology Assessment Group, Department of Health Policy and Management, Harvard University, School of Public Health, F. Mosteller, Director, 677 Huntington Avenue, Boston, MA 02115, 1989.
[6] Thorpe, K. E. and Siegel, J. E., *Journal of the American Medical Association*, Vol. 262, No. 15, 1989, pp. 2114–2118.

John Hedley-Whyte[1]

Anesthesia Vapor Monitoring: Questions To Be Answered

REFERENCE: Hedley-Whyte, J., **"Anesthesia Vapor Monitoring: Questions To Be Answered,"** *Continuous Anesthesia Gas Monitoring, ASTM STP 1090,* J. Hedley-Whyte and P. W. Thompson, Eds., American Society for Testing and Materials, Philadelphia, 1990, pp. 3–6.

ABSTRACT: From 1985 to 1987, according to the Medical Device Reporting System of the United States Food and Drug Administration, 1554 deaths were ascribed to medical devices either wholly or in part; another 29 176 patients were seriously injured. Anesthesia machines were the subject of 1807 malfunction reports during this time and were the medical device sixth most likely to cause death. An award of 15 million dollars was made in the United States for failure to detect a change in anesthetic concentration. Cost of anesthesia vapor monitoring varies, but the costs of additional training in its use have also to be considered. If anesthesia vapor monitoring is to become universal, the versatility of the anesthesia machine and circuit can be cut down.

KEY WORDS: anesthesiology, assessments, design standards, government, medical equipment/medical equipment failure, performance evaluation, standardization

In the standards process one of the first questions is, "Should there be a standard?" When a standard is developed, it has policy implications for practice, cost, and safety. Although the U.S. Government has evidence that anesthesia machines still cause significant mortality (Tables 1, 2, 3, and 4) [1], it is unclear whether work should be started on a standard for continuous anesthetic vapor monitoring. So International Organization for Standardization (ISO) Technical Committee TC 121 and ASTM Committee F-29 decided that one way to resolve this question and therefore advise standards writing bodies, and thus governments, was to have a meeting of experts from academia, from manufacturing, from government, and from standards writing bodies.

The aim of this publication, based on that meeting, was to make a recommendation— either that it is wise or unwise to proceed with the standard. That recommendation will be based on answers to various questions.

The questions obviously are, first, safety: will there be increased safety from what is recommended? This includes safety to the patient, to operating room personnel, and in the widest sense, to our planetary environment. Cost is clearly important. There is cost to the patient, cost to the environment, cost in litigation, and the latter may not be trivial. An award of over 15 million dollars was recently made in the United States for failure to pick up a change in anesthetic concentration.

Cost of anesthesia vapor monitoring equipment varies widely and can be assessed accurately, but one must not forget the cost of additional training. Each time we add equipment or modify medical practice, there is an enormous cost in extra training, which has frequently

[1]David S. Sheridan Professor of Anaesthesia and Respiratory Therapy, Harvard Medical School, and professor in the Department of Health Policy and Management, Harvard School of Public Health, Harvard University, Boston, MA 02115.

TABLE 1—*Overall medical device regulation (MDR) reporting rates by type of report, 1985–1987.*[a]

Type of Report	1985		1986		1987		All 3 years	
	No. of Reports	Percent	No. of Reports	Percent	No. of Reports	Percent	No. of Reports	Percent
Death	561	3	513	3	480	3	1 554	3
Serious injury	9 044	50	11 057	61	9 075	54	29 176	55
Malfunction	8 349	47	6 685	37	7 099	43	22 133	42
Total	17 954	100	18 255	100[b]	16 654	100	52 863	100

[a] From the U.S. General Accounting Office, *Medical Devices: FDA's Implementation of the Medical Device Reporting Regulation* [1].
[b] Percentages do not total 100 because of rounding. Source: MDR data tape provided by FDA.

TABLE 2—*The ten most frequently reported devices, 1985–1987.*[a]

Device Name	No. of Reports	Percent
Pacemaker	14 243	27
Pacemaker electrode	5 304	10
Ventilator	4 115	8
Glucose monitor[b]	1 886	4
Anesthesia machine	1 807	3
Heart valve	1 390	3
Breast prosthesis, inflatable	1 356	3
Infusion pump	1 349	3
Intravascular administration set	972	2
Breast prosthesis, silicone	636	1
Top ten devices	33 058	63[c]
All other devices	19 805	37
Total: all devices	52 863	100

[a] From U.S. General Accounting Office, *Medical Devices: FDA's Implementation of the Medical Device Reporting Regulation* [1].

[b] Includes reports on glucose hexokinase, an in vitro diagnostic reagent used in blood glucose monitoring devices.

[c] Percentages do not add to 63% because of rounding. Source: MDR data tape provided by FDA.

TABLE 3—*The ten devices most frequently reported as associated with the death of patients, 1985–1987.*[a]

Device	No. of Reports	Percent
Heart valve	244	16
Defibrillator	240	15
Pacemaker	90	6
Ventilator	88	6
Pacemaker electrode	60	4
Anesthesia machine	53	3
Intravascular diagnostic catheter	50	3
Infusion pump	47	3
Tampon	40	3
Intra-aortic balloon	24	2
Top ten devices	936	60[b]
All other devices	618	40
Total: all devices	1554	100

[a] From U.S. General Accounting Office, *Medical Devices: FDA's Implementation of the Medical Device Reporting Regulation* [1].

[b] Percentages do not add to 60% because of rounding. Source: MDR data type provided by FDA.

been hidden both from the government and from the general public. We have more medical and paramedical personnel per bed now than 20 years ago. A main reason is because of changes in practice that involve equipment.

If anesthetists are going to move to lower flow anesthesia, they will have to take into account problems of pregnancy, extremes of age, shock, obesity trauma, altitude, abnormal lung function such as chronic obstructive pulmonary disease and asthma, and congestive cardiac failure. All of these have to be considered in the extra training. Most anesthetists are not as familiar with low flow techniques, which tend to follow continuous anesthesia vapor monitoring.

Electrical failure is becoming more common in the Western World. There are still problems with piped oxygen [2] and nitrous oxide [3] supply failure and with compressed gases [4,5]

TABLE 4—*The ten devices most frequently reported as malfunctioning.*

Device Name	No. of Reports	Percent
Ventilator	3 972	18
Pacemaker	2 136	10
Anesthesia machine	1 693	8
Glucose monitor	1 672	8
Infusion pump	980	4
Intravascular administration set	811	4
Pacemaker electrode	805	4
Intra-aortic balloon	517	2
Respiratory gas humidifier	365	2
Peritoneal dialysis administration set, disposable	348	2
Top ten devices	13 299	60[b]
All other devices	8 834	40
Total: all devices	22 133	100

[a] From U.S. General Accounting Office, *Medical Devices: FDA's Implementation of the Medical Device Reporting Regulation* [1].
[b] Percentages do not add to 60 because of rounding. Source: MDR data tape provided by FDA.

from tanks. For medicolegal reasons and reasons of patient care, charting differences frequently have to be overcome. If you do introduce anesthesia vapor monitoring, the versatility of the circuitry can be cut down, and that has pros and cons. Temperature control with low flow anesthesia may be harder, and the early detection of hyperthermia may present problems.

The logistics for remote areas have to be considered because—at least in the United States—there is now evidence that the malpractice burden is one reason for the bankruptcy of remote hospitals, and we are having a lot of bankruptcy of hospitals in the United States at the moment.

References

[1] U.S. General Accounting Office, report to the Chairman, Subcommittee on Health and the Environment, Committee on Energy and Commerce, House of Representatives, "Medical Devices: FDA's Implementation of the Medical Device Reporting Regulation," Report No. GAO/PEMD-89-10, GAO, Washington, DC, 1989.
[2] Feeley, T. W., McClelland, K. J., and Malhotra, I. V., *The Lancet*, Vol. 1, 1975, pp. 1416–1418.
[3] Feeley, T. W. and Hedley-Whyte, J., *Anesthesiology*, Vol. 44, 1976, pp. 301–305.
[4] Eichhorn, J. H., Bancroft, M. L., Laasberg, L. H., du Moulin, G. C., and Saubermann, A. J., *Anesthesiology*, Vol. 46, 1977, pp. 286–289.
[5] Feeley, T. W., Bancroft, M. L., Brooks, R. A., and Hedley-Whyte, J., *Anesthesiology*, Vol. 48, 1978, pp. 72–74.

Charles Whitcher[1]

Volatile Agent Monitoring

REFERENCE: Whitcher, C., **"Volatile Agent Monitoring,"** *Continuous Anesthesia Gas Monitoring, ASTM STP 1090*, J. Hedley-Whyte and P. W. Thompson, Eds., American Society for Testing and Materials, Philadelphia, 1990, pp. 7–19.

ABSTRACT: A case for routine monitoring of volatile anesthetic agents (halocarbons) is based on presumptions of enhanced patient safety, quality patient care, and economy. The patient under anesthesia stands to benefit when halocarbon concentrations in anesthetic gas mixtures are precisely known. Although dial settings of halocarbon vaporizers may roughly approximate halocarbon concentrations present in anesthetic breathing systems, several factors contribute to discrepancies between dial-set concentrations and directly measured concentrations. These discrepancies are often clinically significant. The variables causing discrepancies are complex, being influenced by multiple factors such as the duration of anesthesia, flow rates of gases employed with halocarbons, and vaporizer accuracy. These variables are often difficult to predict and correct for. Therefore, the continuous monitoring of halocarbon concentrations in anesthetic breathing systems offers the most viable method of assessing the halocarbon concentrations present.

Halometry is likely to prove cost-effective on at least two counts, including facilitation of economical reduced flow-rate anesthetic techniques, which conserve expensive halocarbons, and decreased anesthetic mishaps due to over- and underdosage, which may reduce litigation and insurance rates.

Halometers are readily available for routine use. Clinically useful features include frequency response sufficient for breath-by-breath analysis, as end-tidal concentrations are related to anesthetic depth. Readability to two significant figures is also useful. The capability of specific agent recognition seems important primarily when vaporizers are easily misfilled with wrong agents. The overall complexity of patient monitoring need not be objectionably increased by routine halometry. The time may be appropriate for a halometry standard.

KEY WORDS: agents, anesthetics, halocarbons, halometry, monitoring, anesthetic agent monitoring, halocarbon monitoring, halometry, monitoring of anesthetic depth, monitoring of halocarbons, volatile agent monitoring

The objective of this paper is to convey information of possible use in the development of a standard for devices which monitor anesthetic vapors such as isoflurane.

Epidemiology

About 20 000 000 anesthetics are administered annually in the U.S. Estimates of anesthetic deaths range from 2000 to 10 000 per year; 33 to 90% of these deaths are considered preventable. Halocarbons and their vaporizers play a role in deaths considered preventable.

Keenan [1] has reported that 33% of cardiac arrests were caused by absolute agent overdose, defined as dosage of agent above normal clinical concentrations. An additional 33% of cardiac arrests were caused by relative agent overdose, defined as a normal clinical dose which the patient did not tolerate.

The rate of insurance claims paid relative to anesthetic mishaps is about 1.5 per 10 000

---

[1]Professor of anesthesia, Department of Anesthesia, Stanford University School of Medicine, Stanford, CA 94305.

anesthetics, or about one mishap each eight years for an average practice. Although the rate of claims paid is higher than desirable, mishaps are expected infrequently in any individual anesthetist's practice. Thus, based on individual experience, it is difficult to discern whether any given procedure or piece of equipment is either safe or unsafe [2]. For example, the anesthetist may use a copper kettle vaporizer for many years without mishap and therefore conclude, on the basis of personal experience, that this type of vaporizer is safe. On the other hand, the manufacturer bases an impression of safety on the collective experience of many anesthetists. Certain manufacturers perceive that the kettle type vaporizer is frequently implicated in mishaps [3].

Cooper's studies [4] show that 1% of 507 reported critical incidents involved difficulties with vaporizers. Of critical incidents with substantive negative outcomes, overdosage of inhalation agents was involved in 2.9%. Judgemental overdosage figured in 11% of substantive negative outcomes. These results are open to bias because of changes in vaporizer practices during studies. Kettle vaporizers were being phased out, and preventive maintenance programs were newly applied to selected vaporizers. Certain notably imprecise vaporizers were still in use [5].

Mishaps, including those related to halocarbon misdosage, may appear to occur randomly, involving even the most experienced, conscientious anesthetist and even the healthiest, lowest risk patient. Although the higher ASA physical status classes of patients are the most at risk on a per patient basis, the lower ASA physical status classes are the most frequently anesthetized. By reason of their larger numbers, and neglecting their presumably greater physiologic stability, the latter group may be the more at risk and therefore the more likely to benefit from monitoring.

Outpatients appear to be at substantially lower risk than inpatients, with the former showing anesthetic mortality rates of 1:50 000 [6] versus 1:5000 to 1:10 000, respectively. Reasons for the lower rate remain to be shown. However, outpatients are generally younger and healthier, and the types of surgical procedures performed are usually less complicated. Their apparently lower mortality could possibly be considered as an indication for a somewhat lesser level of monitoring than in the case of inpatients. However, avoidable risks must be held to a minimum, and the breath-by-breath monitoring of all ventilatory gases and vapors among all patients may be presumed to maximize patient safety.

Mishaps and Their Prevention: Monitoring

Frequently recurrent mishaps, together with monitors designed to recognize them, are shown in Figure 1. Categories of mishaps shown which may involve halocarbons and vaporizers primarily include overdosage and underdosage. Insufficient halocarbon may be associated with hyperventilation, hypertension, and tachycardia, arrythmias, and recall. Overdosage may cause hypoventilation, hypotension, and cardiac arrest.

The clinical utility of monitoring with sophisticated equipment such as the halometer is not to be minimized, but the use of such equipment represents a supplement to, not a substitute for, good clinical judgement and basic direct clinical observations. The primary protection against mishaps is the alert, attentive, well-trained clinician, continuously observing the patient and the anesthesia equipment with the unaided senses. Elaborate monitoring miscarries if it becomes a distraction.

Although a significant component of clinical anesthesia remains an art tempered by clinical judgement, anesthetic practice is becoming increasingly quantitative as rapidly improving instruments become available. It is now technically simple to measure the concentrations of each gas ventilated by the patient, breath by breath, at a level of precision which is comparable with the usual precise administration of intravenous drugs. Although the unaided senses play an important role in monitoring, the patient may be inaccessible to direct observations. Surgical draping may almost completely cover the patient, particularly in

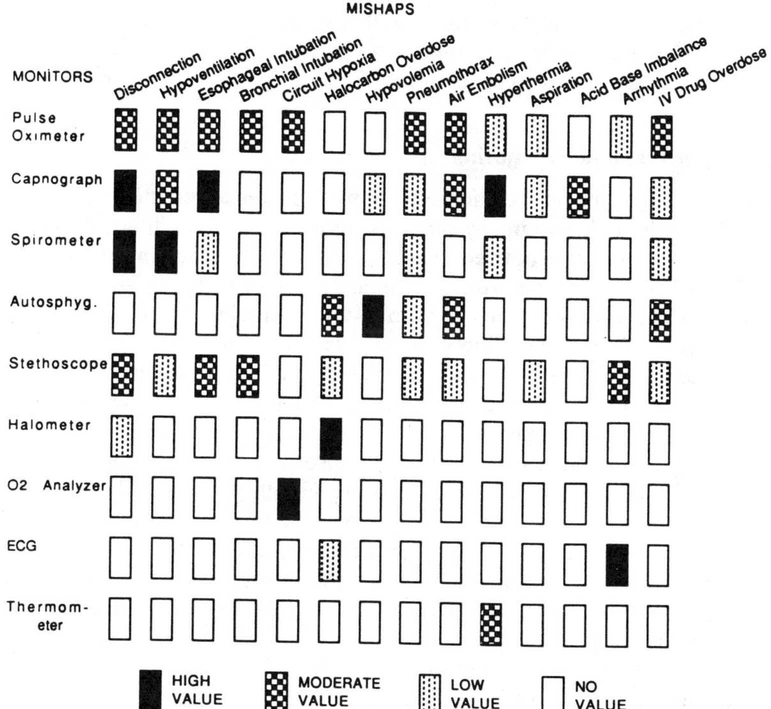

FIG. 1—*Matrix of monitoring equipment versus type of mishap. This matrix represents the author's estimate of the most useful monitors in mishap prevention. A nerve stimulator for assessment of neuromuscular blockade would be added to a list of most useful routine monitors. IV = intravenous; Autosphygmomanometer = automatic noninvasive sphygmomanometer; 02 analyzer = breathing circuit oxygen analyzer; ECG = monitor of cardiac electrical activity. Adapted (with permission) from: Whitcher C., Ream A. K., Parsons D., et al., "Anesthetic Mishaps and the Cost of Monitoring: A Proposed Standard for Monitoring Equipment,* Journal of Clinical Monitoring, *Vol. 4, 1988, pp. 5–15.*

certain plastic, eye, ear, nose and throat, and neurosurgical procedures, maximizing the need for instrumental monitoring aid. Moreover, instruments can measure physiologic functions which cannot be directly observed, e.g., end-tidal concentrations of halocarbons. A further advantage is the alarms provided by monitors, which, when well designed, can alert the anesthetist when attention must be directed away from direct patient observations. Alarms provide early warning, gaining time to muster corrective measures and indicating the success of those measures.

How may the incidence of mishaps be reduced? Continuing efforts are in order to improve resident selection and to offer enhanced training programs both during residency and continuing thereafter. The critical importance of vigilance is obvious. The development of simulators is promising. However, it seems unrealistic to expect substantial improvement in human factors such as resident selection and training, and in vigilance. On the other hand, the rapid improvements in monitoring, including halometry, could reasonably lead to a reduction of mishaps.

The author's case for routine halometry is based on presumptions of enhanced patient safety, quality of patient care, continuing education of the anesthetist, and economy. Mishaps due to unexpected concentrations of halocarbons, both high and low, may be prevented. The quality of patient care and the continuing education of the anesthetist may both be enhanced with the anesthetist continuously informed of the precise inhaled and end-tidal concentrations of halocarbons, breath by breath. Economy may be achievable through the use of low flow-rate anesthetic techniques, facilitated by monitoring, and by mishap prevention, which leads to reductions of insurance claims paid and insurance rates.

Halocarbon Vaporizers and Monitoring

Halocarbon vaporizers may be considered as sensitive halocarbon metering devices serving life-supporting anesthetic breathing systems. A noticeable, often clinically significant, discrepancy nearly always prevails between concentrations of halocarbons in breathing systems predicted from dial settings of vaporizers, compared with directly measured concentrations. Multiple, complex factors are involved, such as the accuracy of vaporizers, flow rates of gases employed with halocarbons, time-varying uptake rates of halocarbons, cardiac output, and variations in pulmonary ventilation. Vaporizers occasionally run dry. Depending on the law of mass action or the relative concentrations of halocarbon in the patient and in the breathing circuit, the patient may absorb agent from, or elute agent into, the breathing circuit. During anesthetic induction, when agent absorption is rapid, both inhaled and end-tidal agent concentrations in breathing circuits are usually considerably below the dial-set concentration of the vaporizer. During recovery, when the vaporizer is turned off, the inhaled concentrations of agent rapidly approaches zero, while agent eluting from the patient reduces much more slowly with time. Continuous monitoring offers the most viable method of coping with the multiple, complex causes of divergencies between vaporizer settings and concentrations actually present.

Vaporizers are rarely in perfect calibration. A 1985 study of vaporizer accuracy [7] shows that measured concentrations of halocarbons may be at least twice, to less than half, of dial set concentrations. A vaporizer known to be accurate, defined as delivering plus or minus 10% of dial-set concentrations, sent out for routine maintenance and calibration, was returned delivering isoflurane 2.7% at a dial setting of isoflurane 1.0%. Kettle-type vaporizers performed no better than agent-specific calibrated vaporizers, probably because of flow meter inaccuracy. Modern vaporizers were usually more accurate than older units, within plus or minus 20% of dial settings. Many obsolescent, inaccurate vaporizers remain in regular clinical use.

Other factors which may result in unexpected halocarbon concentrations are found in obsolescent anesthetic equipment. A vaporizer on-off switch may be inconspicuous and mistakenly either on or off. A missing vaporizer filler plug or stopper key may vent vaporized halocarbon and gases, including oxygen, to room air. A movable vaporizer may have been recently tipped, yielding very high halocarbon concentrations.

A human variable involving obsolescent equipment is the vintage of the anesthetist's training. The more recent the training, the less the familiarity with features and hazards of obsolescent equipment. Kettle-type vaporizers easily deliver lethal concentrations of halocarbons. A resident may never use a kettle during training, yet in practice a kettle alone may be available. Again, halometry offers protection; alarms give early warning.

Halometers

Criteria of an ideal monitor for use in anesthesia are: It must be informative of patient condition, highly reliable and easy to use, free of misleading artifacts, and economical. Several categories of monitors which meet these criteria are readily available for the clinical measurement of halocarbons. Long-established methods depend on the principles of mass and infrared spectroscopies. Raman effect and piezoelectric monitors are also available. A photoacoustic monitor has recently become available.

Stand Alone Versus Time-Shared Halometers

Mass spectrometer systems which have been available since about 1979 are intended for time-shared use. A single mass spectrometer unit is implemented with a computer-controlled valve for receiving samples from each room in sequence. A long sampling line from each room receives sample gases from each breathing circuit. Results of analysis are reported on a display device in each room. Disadvantages of this type of system are widespread loss of comprehensive monitoring in case of system breakdown, and delay in reporting. By sampling each room for 20 s, a 16-bed operating room would expect updated data about every 5 min. It has been recommended that a single mass spectrometer should serve no more than eight rooms. The impact of loss of monitoring in case of system breakdown may be attenuated by supplemental equipment. The two U.S. sources of central mass spectrometer systems offer a supplemental infrared capnometer which continuously displays the carbon dioxide wave form on the cathode ray tube, independent of the mass spectrometer and computer. An advantage of a central system is centralized calibration. A further possible advantage is economy, in that comprehensive gas analysis may be provided at lower cost than in the case of certain stand-alone monitors.

A recently developed stand-alone mass spectrometer (Ohmeda) may be commended for its compact size, easy mobility, low sampling flow rate (30 mL/min), and well-designed display and alarms. A recently developed Raman analyzer (Albion) is promising. Both units specifically analyze all gases and vapors usually associated with anesthesia.

Agent Specificity

Most of the infrared halometers available at writing must be manually programmed for the specific halocarbon in use. A single wave length of infrared light is used for analysis. However, by using multiple wavelengths of infrared light, specific halocarbons can be recognized. A generation of monitors with this capability is expected in the near future.

An ideal halometer would be capable of quantitating any specific halocarbon in any volatile anesthetic mixture. Whether the extra instrumental complexity involved is worthwhile may depend on the filling systems of halocarbon vaporizers available in a given suite of operating rooms. Simple pour-filled vaporizers are easily misfilled with wrong agents. On the other hand, a high level of protection against unexpected liquid agent mixtures is provided by keyed vaporizer-filling systems, readily available with modern vaporizers. Such systems key each specific halocarbon bottle to each halocarbon-specific vaporizer. The author is aware of no reports of substantive patient injury due to unrecognized mixtures of halocarbons.

Frequency Response

The issue of instrument frequency response is clinically relevant and important to consider in any standards writing. Halothane is a notably weak absorber of infrared light at wavelengths usually employed in halometers. Therefore, this agent is the most difficult to measure, relative to other halocarbons, and must therefore govern critical design features which provide for adequate frequency response. The frequency response of many capnometers approaches a range of 100 to 200 ms, while that of certain infrared halometers approaches a range of 600 to 800 ms. The author's limited studies [7] suggest that a 600-ms response is clinically useful, particularly under near-equilibrium conditions when the breath-by-breath changes of halocarbon concentrations amount to only a few tenths of 1%. When concentrations are changing markedly and rapidly, some rounding of waveform angles is likely to occur. If instrumental standards are to be written, requirements of frequency response should be carefully investigated.

Significant Figures

Readability to two significant figures is a clinically useful feature of halometers, particularly in the 0 to 1% range. This feature is not available in most modern instruments. Manufacturers indicate that two-decimal-place accuracy is difficult to achieve in such a range, particularly in the case of halothane. This granted, the clinician is more concerned with slight changes of concentrations than with absolute accuracy, as detailed later under clinical notes.

Halometry and Complexity of Monitoring

It may be argued that halometry, if added to the list of required monitors, could unduly contribute to the complexity of monitoring and saddle the anesthetist with one more ill-affordable distraction. Obviously, each additional monitor can only add some measure of complexity. If a new monitor is to be adopted, the additional burden imposed should be more than compensated by the usefulness of the data provided.

Capnometry, an evolving standard, is increasingly available. Given a capnometer which obtains samples via catheter, the most prevalent type, the addition of a halometer imposes only a minimal additional burden for the following reasons:

1. *Components of the two monitors may be shared.* Obvious components which may be shared include the airway adapter, sampling catheter, sampling pump, and sample disposal line [7]. The two monitors are best combined in a single case.

2. *The halographic waveform need not necessarily be displayed.* With the capnographic waveform displayed (an essential component of capnometry, in the opinion of many), the halographic data may be displayed in numeric format alone. Given a properly designed halometer with adequate frequency response, the capnogram alone may be sufficient to verify appropriate sampling.

3. *Interpretation of the halogram is simple, relative to the capnogram.* The capnogram is influenced by breathing circuit, ventilatory, cardiovascular, and metabolic considerations. Accordingly, interpretation is complex. Although multiple factors also influence the halogram, the displayed values are usually used primarily for the precise measurement of inhaled and end-tidal concentrations, and as a guide to supplement the clinician's judgement in the setting of flow meters and vaporizer to sustain the desired depth of anesthesia.

Artifacts

Any monitor is potentially capable of presenting artifacts and inaccurate, misleading information. Instrument maintenance and calibration must be appropriate. The anesthetist must be familiar with the features of the monitor and its requirements for proper use. Limitations, always present, must be understood.

Sampling Techniques

In the case of halometry, as in capnometry, the sampling technique is critical in obtaining interpretable results. Assuming that the capnogram alone is displayed, the quality of the capnogram may be taken to indicate the quality of the halogram. The capnogram must show sharply defined end-tidal plateaus and returns to baseline. Samples must be obtained sufficiently close to a point of to-and-fro rebreathing within the patient's airway in order to avoid sample dilution by fresh gases from the breathing circuit or room air. Sampling becomes increasingly difficult as tidal volumes reduce and ventilatory rates increase. Suboptimal sampling is unacceptable when misleading information is obtained. The expected sharp corners of the ideal wave shape may be blunted, and plateaus, although present, may fall short of the actual end-tidal data.

Among small patients, especially neonates, sampling is critical and may require specialized apparatus. A special 15-mm endotracheal tube adapter with built-in side port for sampling usually suffices for infants and small children (Fig. 2). In the case of neonates, the best results are apt to be achieved using a special endotracheal tube with built-in sampling catheter. Samples are obtained at the distal beveled end of the endotracheal tube. Occlusion with secretions might be anticipated, but the author's experience is that this problem is surprisingly rare in the operating room.

Sampling technique must be especially meticulous when modified Mapleson D (Bain) type breathing systems are employed. There is the possibility of dilution of sample gases by the fresh gas stream. Waveforms may seem appropriate, but the height of capnometric and halometric plateaus may be artifactually reduced, yielding inconspicuously misleading information. The suggested special sampling equipment is usually compatible with appropriate data.

Sampling may be the most uncritical among adult patients with large tidal volumes and low ventilatory rates. Even with face mask techniques, interpretable information may be obtained by sampling at the Y-piece of the circle breathing circuit. However, if dead space within the mask is large relative to the tidal volume, waveforms may be uninterpretable. Improvement is likely to be achieved by sampling at a site 1 cm within a patent naris, or from an oral or nasopharyngeal airway.

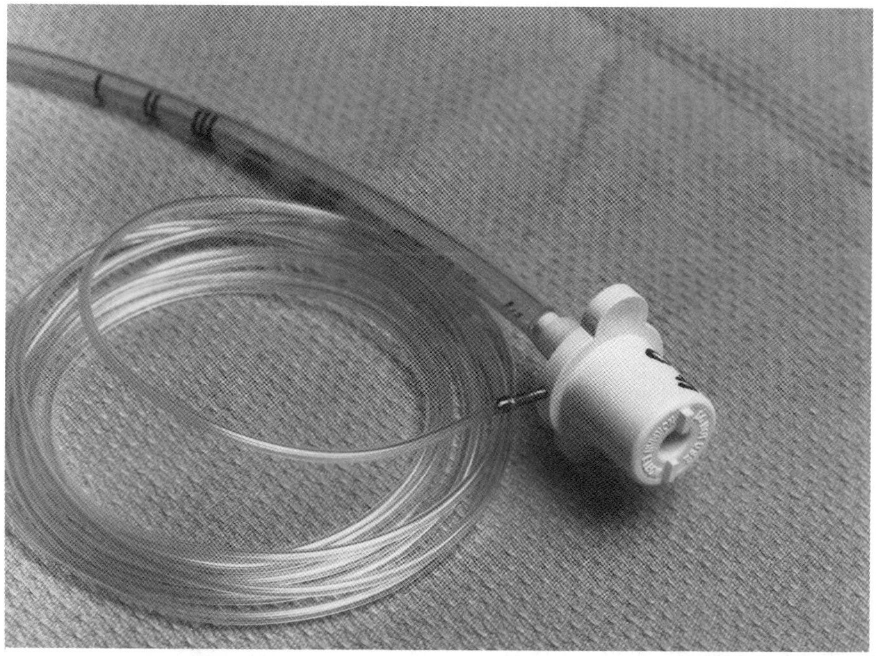

FIG. 2—*15-mm pediatric endotracheal tube adapter with sampling port. Lumen of sampling catheter opens into airway. Thick adapter wall minimizes deadspace. Caution: Certain pediatric breathing circuits may not fit minimal deadspace adapters. Adapted (with permission) from: Whitcher C. "Monitoring of Anesthetic Halocarbons: Self-Contained ('Stand Alone') Equipment,"* Seminars in Anesthesia, *Vol. 5, 1986, pp. 213–224.*

Halography

The following waveforms and interpretations provided are intended to elucidate the clinical significance of inhaled and end-tidal halocarbon data.

Figure 3 shows short strips of the simultaneously recorded waveforms of carbon dioxide and isoflurane, recorded at a paper speed sufficient to show waveform details. Three representative periods of anesthesia are shown, including induction, maintenance, and recovery (A, B, and C, respectively). Capnographic waveforms appear above, halographic waveforms below. The capnogram is represented to verify appropriate sampling, i.e., sharply defined end-tidal plateaus and returns to baseline, and as a marker of inhalation and exhalation. Exhalation is approximately marked by the end-tidal plateau, inhalation approximately by the baseline.

Referring to Figure 3A, inhaled concentrations of isoflurane represent isoflurane present in the breathing circuit. End-tidal concentrations represent alveolar concentrations, which, under equilibrium conditions, indicate tissue concentrations. Tissue concentrations offer some indication of depth of anesthesia, although anesthetic depth is a complex modality influenced by multiple factors including premedication, surgical requirements, etc. During induction, the patient absorbs agent rapidly, so that a considerable difference is notable between inhaled and end-tidal concentrations.

Among clinical implications, if end-tidal concentrations of halocarbons are inadequate, the unparalyzed patient will move when stimulated. During the induction of anesthesia, there is often a conflict of interest between the maintenance of adequate blood pressure and adequate end-tidal halocarbon concentrations. Prior to surgical stimulation, hypotension is a recurrent concern.

Referring to Figure 3B, the maintenance phase of anesthesia, under the more nearly steady-state conditions of the maintenance phase, the inhaled and end-tidal halocarbon concentrations are more nearly alike. The patient absorbs halocarbon more slowly relative to the induction phase. However, even in the case of prolonged anesthesia, a perceptible inhaled/exhaled difference persists because saturation never becomes complete during the course of anesthesia.

If, during maintenance, the vaporizer setting is changed sufficiently, the difference between inhaled and exhaled concentrations quickly increases because near-equilibrium conditions are upset. If the vaporizer setting is increased, inhaled concentrations suddenly increase. If the vaporizer setting is decreased sufficiently, end-tidal concentrations exceed inhaled concentrations since the patient becomes the predominating source of isoflurane in the breathing circuit.

Among clinical implications of halometry during maintenance, the end-tidal measurement provides a quantitative, reproducible measurement of a relationship to level of anesthesia, relative to the halocarbon employed. A narcotic may be used either to supplement the halocarbon, or as the primary agent, with halocarbon supplementation. Given end-tidal measurements of halocarbon, tissue levels, although not measured, are assumed to be maintained at desired concentrations. Tissue concentrations are usually somewhat lower than end-tidal concentrations.

Referring to Figure 3C, the recovery phase of anesthesia, the vaporizer is off, the patient is the primary source of isoflurane, and end-tidal concentrations are higher than inhaled concentrations.

Since halocarbons are highly soluble in body tissues, end-tidal concentrations diminish more slowly as the duration of anesthesia increases. It is usually difficult to arouse a patient if end-tidal concentrations are as high as 0.3%. On the other hand, there is a good chance that the patient will awaken as concentrations approach 0.2%. The trends between 0.3 and 0.2% are thus important and best observable in monitors with scales which are readable to

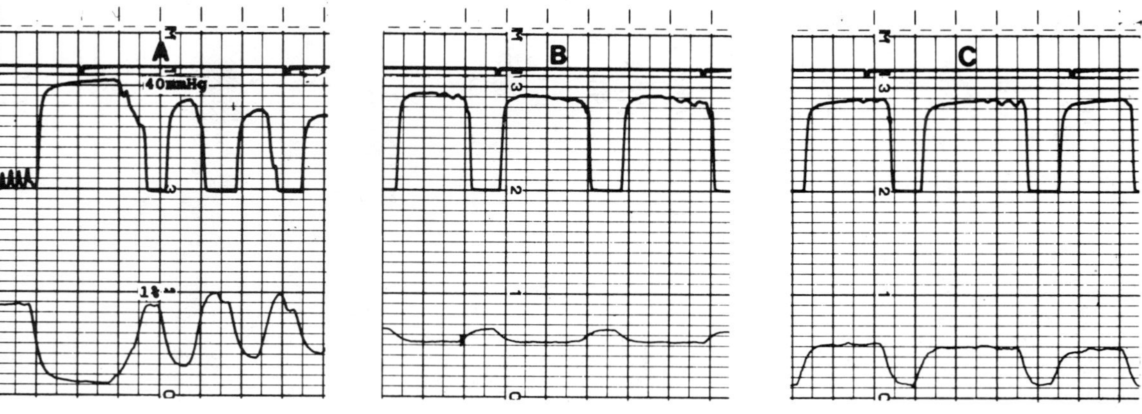
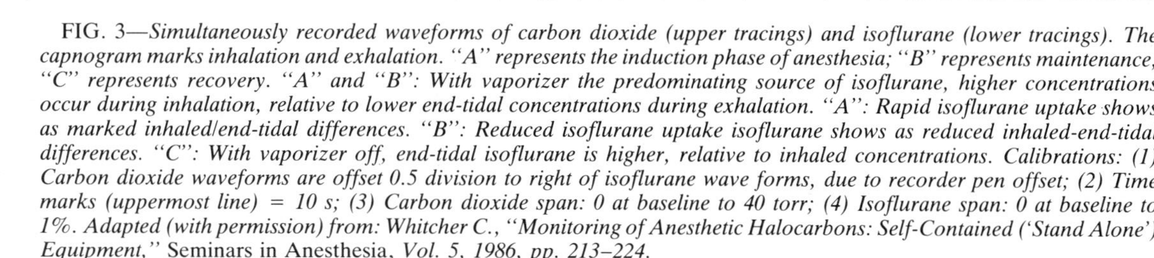

FIG. 3—*Simultaneously recorded waveforms of carbon dioxide (upper tracings) and isoflurane (lower tracings). The capnogram marks inhalation and exhalation. "A" represents the induction phase of anesthesia; "B" represents maintenance; "C" represents recovery. "A" and "B": With vaporizer the predominating source of isoflurane, higher concentrations occur during inhalation, relative to lower end-tidal concentrations during exhalation. "A": Rapid isoflurane uptake shows as marked inhaled/end-tidal differences. "B": Reduced isoflurane uptake isoflurane shows as reduced inhaled-end-tidal differences. "C": With vaporizer off, end-tidal isoflurane is higher, relative to inhaled concentrations. Calibrations: (1) Carbon dioxide waveforms are offset 0.5 division to right of isoflurane wave forms, due to recorder pen offset; (2) Time marks (uppermost line) = 10 s; (3) Carbon dioxide span: 0 at baseline to 40 torr; (4) Isoflurane span: 0 at baseline to 1%. Adapted (with permission) from: Whitcher C., "Monitoring of Anesthetic Halocarbons: Self-Contained ('Stand Alone') Equipment," Seminars in Anesthesia, Vol. 5, 1986, pp. 213–224.*

two significant figures. Absolute accuracy is always desirable among monitors, but the capability of observing direction of change is even more desirable.

Figure 4 shows a halometer tracing for an entire case recorded at slow speed to show trends, with waveform details not discernable. During the induction of anesthesia (left), the vaporizer is turned up sufficiently to yield inhaled isoflurane concentrations of about 2.5%, represented by the upward pointed peak values of waveforms. The minimum values of the induction waveforms, representing end-tidal concentrations, describe the uptake curve of isoflurane. Slightly to the right, the inhaled concentrations instantly diminish to isoflurane about 1.2%, marking a reduction of vaporizer setting, accompanied by end-tidal concentrations of isoflurane about 0.8%. Minor vaporizer adjustments are apparent during the main part of the case, reflected in limited but sharply defined changes of inhaled concentrations, these accompanied by more limited changes in end-tidal concentrations. At the end of the case (right), the vaporizer is turned off, marked by an abrupt reduction of inhaled concentrations. Waveform detail is not shown, but this reduction instantly reaches baseline, while end-tidal concentrations slowly reduce, never quite reaching zero. The patient became rousable, however, when isoflurane reached about 0.2%.

An Economic Issue and Low Flow-Rate Techniques

Incentives to reduce the cost of patient care are increasing. Modern halocarbons are expensive; costs may be substantially reduced through the use of low flow-rate techniques. Such techniques have been available for a long time, but utilization remains limited; prevailing training programs continue to emphasize high flow-rate techniques. One reason is the perceived technical ease and safety of high flow-rate techniques and the relative complexity of low flow-rate techniques. Halometry may substantially simplify the use of low flow rates.

In a conventional high flow-rate circle carbon dioxide absorption technique, typical flow-meter settings are nitrous oxide at 3 L/min and oxygen at 2 L/min, supplemented with isoflurane at 1% from the vaporizer. These flow rates represent large excesses, since the

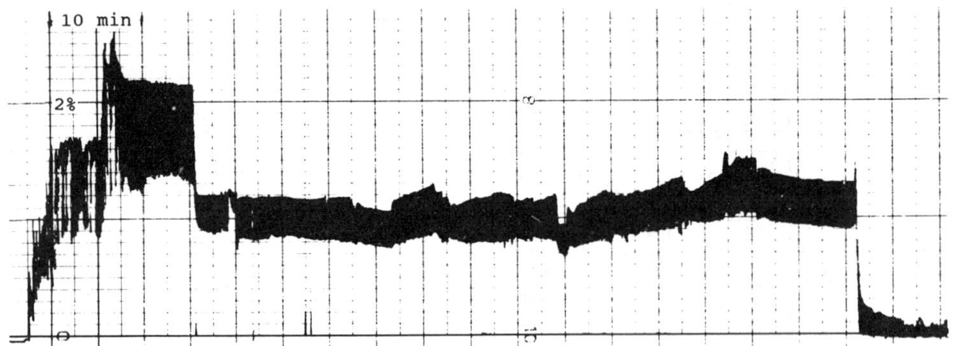

FIG. 4—*Slow-speed tracing of isoflurane showing events and trends. Induction and recovery (extreme left and main center section): End-tidal concentrations are the lower concentrations. Recovery (extreme right): End-tidal concentrations are the higher concentrations. With induction, vaporizer is set at high concentrations; end-tidal concentrations increase slowly. Abrupt changes in upper inhaled concentrations result when vaporizer settings are changed. During maintenance, minor vaporizer adjustments result in minor changes of inhaled and end-tidal concentrations. During recovery, end-tidal (upper) concentrations diminish slowly. Waking is expected at a certain low concentration, e.g. isoflurane 0.2% to 0.3%, depending on adjuvent medications. Calibrations: (1) Time: 2.5 min. per vertical line; (2) Isoflurane: 0 baseline—2%. Adapted (with permission) from: Whitcher C., "Monitoring of Anesthetic Halocarbons: Self-Contained ('Stand Alone') Equipment," Seminars in Anesthesia, Vol. 5, 1986, pp. 213–224.*

patient absorbs oxygen at about 200 cc/min, nitrous oxide at about 50 cc/min, and isoflurane at about 15 cc/min. Because of the excess, the composition of the gas/vapor mixture is roughly similar anywhere measured, whether in the fresh gas mixture or in the breathing circuit. In other words, the absorption of gases and halocarbon by the patient is inconsequential relative to the large excesses provided. In short, the technique is simple and easy to use. The most obvious disadvantage is costliness: 90% of expensive isoflurane used is nonessential for anesthesia.

In a low flow-rate circle carbon dioxide absorption technique, e.g., nitrous oxide and oxygen at 0.25 L/min each, rebreathing and patient absorption increase the concentration of nitrous oxide above the 50% delivered at the flow meters. The amount of increase varies with time as full saturation with nitrous oxide is approached. Oxygen absorption usually holds constant. Since gas concentrations are easily predictable only within wide limits, adjustments are best made on the basis of monitored concentrations.

The above principles, relative to nitrous oxide in a circle rebreathing system, are equally as applicable to a halocarbon, except that, because of the markedly greater solubility of such an agent in the body compared with nitrous oxide, the effects of time and relative absorption rates of gases are much greater. During the induction of anesthesia, a halocarbon vaporizer setting of 5% may be barely sufficient. Later in the case, with absorption continuing because saturation is never approached, the vaporizer setting may have to be kept at 2 to 3% in order to support an end-tidal halocarbon concentration of 1%.

Although the absorption rates of halocarbons may be calculated on the basis of the square root of time [8], most anesthetists do not use such calculations. The direct measurement of halocarbon concentrations is easier and eliminates possible errors due to miscalculations or variabilities among patients that are not necessarily easy to recognize or to take into account. In other words, halometry facilitates low flow-rate techniques.

Table 1 shows a comparison of the cost of gases and soda lime at high flow-rate and low flow-rate techniques using isoflurane. It is apparent that materials for a 2-h, 5-L/min technique cost $15.41/h, whereas materials for a reduced flow-rate technique cost only $5.63/h.

TABLE 1—*Cost of gases and soda lime related to gas flow rates.*

Assumptions:
1. 2 h average case duration.
2. Isoflurane employed with N_2O, O_2, and soda lime.

| | | High Flow Technique | | | | Low Flow Technique | | | |
Stage	Gas/ Agent	Conc., %	Flow, L/min	Time, min	Cost, $	Conc., %	Flow, L/min	Time, min	Cost, $
Preoxygenation,	O_2		5	2	$ 0.001		5	2	$ 0.001
Intubation	N_2O		0		$ 0.000		0		$ 0.000
	Iso.	0			$ 0.000	0			$ 0.000
Induction (early)	O_2		2	5	$ 0.001		2	5	$ 0.001
	N_2O		3		$ 0.002		3		$ 0.002
	Iso.	2			$ 1.197	2			$ 1.197
Induction (late)	O_2		2	10	$ 0.003		0.5	10	$ 0.001
	N_2O		3		$ 0.005		0.5		$ 0.001
	Iso.	1.5			$ 1.795	3			$ 0.718
Maintenance	O_2		2	103	$ 0.027		0.3	103	$ 0.004
	N_2O		3		$ 0.049		0.2		$ 0.003
	Iso.	1			$12.326	3			$ 3.698
	Soda Lime				$ 0.005				$ 0.420
					Total Cost $ 15.41				Total Cost $ 5.63

Last year, about $140 000 worth of isoflurane was used in the 14 operating rooms of a major medical center, in which this agent was used mostly at high flow rates and primarily as a supplement in balanced techniques with narcotics.

A stand-alone mass spectrometer or Raman analyzer is listed at about $18 000, while infrared and piezoelectric monitors cost $3000 to $15 000. It has been suggested that any such monitors may be cost-effective in the sense that they may reduce mishaps and the consequent cost of litigation and insurance [2].

Notes on the Clinical Use of Low Flow-Rate Techniques

If low flow rates are to be employed, several considerations are relevant. Most modern anesthesia machines are factory adjusted to deliver no less than 0.250 to 0.5 L/min of oxygen, so that the anesthesia machine to be employed at low flow rates may have to be specially adjusted to deliver appropriately reduced flow rates of oxygen. Cases selected at first might best be straightforward and sufficiently long, at least 30 min. The use of a breath-by-breath halometer is assumed. The anesthetist should be familiar with important details in sampling techniques, particularly in the monitoring of infants and neonates.

As rules of thumb:

1. Make breathing system tight, e.g., leakage rate less than 200 cc/min at an in-circuit pressure of 30-cm water. Tightness is always desirable and especially important at low flow rates. Sufficient gas must invariably be retained in breathing circuits; rebreathing bags and bellows must be kept appropriately full.

2. Start case at the high flow rate of choice, e.g., oxygen at 5 L/min.

3. Continue case after intubation with nitrous oxide 3 L/min with oxygen at 2 L/min and end-tidal isoflurane concentrations of 0.5 to 1.5% (vaporizer settings of 1 to 3%), depending on patient responses. Ten minutes into the case, reduce flow meter settings to nitrous and oxygen, 0.5 L/min each, with end-tidal isoflurane concentrations sustained at 0.5 to 1.5% (vaporizer settings of 1 to 4%).

4. Twenty minutes into the case, assuming stable conditions, reduce flow rates to 0.25 L/min each of nitrous oxide and oxygen, with end-tidal isoflurane held to 0.5 to 1.5% (vaporizer settings again 1 to 4%). At the latter flow rates, vaporizer settings may require fine adjustments in order to sustain desired end tidal halocarbon concentrations.

5. In case of any difficulty with the patient, increase flow rates of gases, usually after reducing vaporizer settings. High flow-rate techniques are desirable in their requirement of minimal attention. The importance of reducing vaporizer settings when converting to high flow rates deserves emphasis. If total flow rates of nitrous oxide and oxygen of 0.25 L/min each, at a vaporizer setting of isoflurane 4%, are suddenly increased, the concomitant increase of end-tidal isoflurane rapidly results in halocarbon overdosage.

6. If oxygen concentrations increase above desired levels, slightly reduce the oxygen flow rate, and slightly increase the nitrous oxide flow rate, maintaining the same total gas flow rate. A constant total gas flow rate favors stability of vaporizer output, hence stability of end tidal halocarbon concentrations.

7. If oxygen concentration reduces below desired levels, slightly increase oxygen flow rate, and slightly decrease nitrous oxide flow rate.

8. Note three caveats of low flow-rate techniques:

a. Sustain oxygen always at safe concentrations.

b. Keep sufficient gases in the rebreathing bag or bellows at all time.

c. Check, and usually reduce, vaporizer settings when converting from low flow-rate to high flow-rate techniques.

In the author's training program, most residents find that low flow-rate techniques stimulate a high level of understanding of gas uptake and distribution. Interest and vigilence in long, uneventful cases tends to be sustained. Significant conservation of expensive halocarbons is potentially achievable.

Factors Possibly Retarding Halometry as a Routine Measurement

Halometry is not yet a widespread practice. Several factors may tend to retard general use of the technique. The most obvious factor is that many anesthetists have not yet perceived the advantages. In fact, it is very difficult to appreciate the utility of any new monitor or any unfamiliar technique in the abstract without direct, personal experience in its use. Another factor is inertia. Familiar, proven, comfortable practices tend to persist. Humans tend to believe that what they are doing today is working safely and satisfactorily, so that change is not called for. Since it may be uncomfortable to realize that there could be viable alternatives, any tendency to perceive the need for change may be unconsciously suppressed. There may be an intimidation factor, the fear that the new monitor or unfamiliar method will be difficult to master or may embarrass the anesthetist by an appearance of ineptness during the learning process. Another factor is the leader-follower trait, which causes some to wait while others initiate the use of an alternative method. A final problem is that the anesthetist may not be cost conscious and therefore fail to perceive the need to conserve materials such as expensive halocarbons. As a suggestion, if the hospital administrator were to allocate part of any savings achieved to new anesthetic equipment or other perk, the cooperation of anesthetists might be increased.

Conclusions

The question of need for a standard is obviously complex. Instrumental support for routine halometry is readily available. Inhaled and exhaled concentrations of all gases and halocarbons involved in clinical anesthesia are readily measured. Halometry does not necessarily impose a significant increase in the complexity of monitoring, while offering advantages in enhanced patient safety and quality patient care through the quantitative measurement of halocarbons. Even neglecting the potential savings of reduced flow-rate anesthetic techniques, the cost of halometry appears to be managable and probably cost-effective in terms of anticipated reductions of anesthetic mishaps due to misdosage, and reduced consequent litigation. A halocarbon monitoring standard could well prove to be appropriate.

References

[1] Keenan, R. L. and Boyen, C. P., "Cardiac Arrest Due to Anesthesia," *JAMA*, Vol. 253, 1985, pp. 2373–2377.

[2] Whitcher, C., Ream, R. K., Parsons, D., et al., "Anesthetic Mishaps and the Cost of Monitoring: a Proposed Standard for Monitoring Equipment," *Journal of Clinical Monitoring*, Vol. 4, 1988, pp. 5–15.

[3] Potakar, A. L., "Discussion on Vaporizers," Committee on Education and Training, Anesthesia Patient Safety Foundation, Washington, DC, 24 May 1987.

[4] Cooper, J. B., Newbower, R. S., and Kitz, R. J., "An Analysis of Major Errors and Equipment Failures in Anesthesia Management: Considerations for Prevention and Detection," *Anesthesiology*, Vol. 60, 1984, pp. 34–42.

[5] Hedley-Whyte, J., discussion of Dr. Whitcher's paper, "Volatile Agent Monitoring," meeting of ASTM Committee F-29 on Anesthetic and Respiratory Equipment, 21 February 1989, London.

[6] Keenan, R., "Anesthetic Disasters: Incidence, Causes, Preventability," 38th Annual Refresher Course Lecture Program, 1987 Annual Meeting, American Society of Anesthesiologists, Park Ridge, IL, 11 October 1987.

[7] Whitcher, C., "Monitoring of Anesthetic Halocarbons: Self Contained ('Stand-Alone') Equipment," *Seminars in Anesthesia*, Vol. 5, 1986, pp. 213–224.

[8] Lowe, H. J. and Earnst, E., *The Quantitative Practice of Anesthesia. Use of Closed Circuit*, Williams and Wilkens, Baltimore, 1981.

Markku P. J. Paloheimo[1]

Clinical Aspects of Anesthesia Gas Monitoring

REFERENCE: Paloheimo, M. P. J., **"Clinical Aspects of Anesthesia Gas Monitoring,"** *Continuous Anesthesia Gas Monitoring, ASTM STP 1090*, J. Hedley-Whyte and P. W. Thompson, Eds., American Society for Testing and Materials, Philadelphia, 1990, pp. 20–25.

ABSTRACT: Monitoring of both inspired and end-tidal concentrations of oxygen, carbon dioxide, nitrous oxide, and volatile anesthetic vapors is nowadays possible with a stand-alone unit based on infrared and paramagnetic technologies (Capnomac, Datex/Instrumentarium, Helsinki, Finland). The clinical value of the breath-by-breath information on the management of low-flow and partial rebreathing breathing circuits during various phases of general anesthesia are discussed in the light of multigas trends. It is concluded that quantitative analysis of both gases and halocarbon vapors is informative of gas delivery, uptake, and distribution, provides useful information on patient management, and enhances patient safety.

KEY WORDS: monitoring, physiologic, oxygen, carbon dioxide, nitrous oxide, anesthesia, inhalational, anesthesia, closed circuit

Clinical Aspects of Anesthesia Gas Monitoring

In the anesthesia machine, a gas mixture is prepared that normally becomes the "anesthetic fresh gas" and is fed into the anesthesia circuit [1]. There are many factors that affect the final concentration of the gas mixture administered as a tidal volume to the patient. These factors include the fresh gas flow, the circuit volume, the expiratory gas composition, and the order of the components in the circuit itself [2]. Expiratory gas mixture, and its last portion, in particular, reflects the alveolar concentrations of the gases, which is the step in the oxygen cascade that is met by pulmonary circulation. Alveolar concentrations are influenced by other, often unpredictable factors, such as cardiac output, specific gas solubility in blood, and peripheral uptake from the blood, which determines the concentration gradients between the venous blood and the alveoli. The most comprehensive information is available from the patient Y-piece, where both inspiratory and end-tidal gas concentrations can be measured, rather than by monitoring the output of the anesthesia machine. Monitoring of all the gases normally used during general anesthesia may be beneficial to the patient.

The patient is normally preoxygenated prior to the induction of anesthesia. Figure 1 shows a trend of the end-tidal oxygen concentration, where the face mask is held 5 cm above the face and 3 min later lowered to touch the face, although not kept tight. In a modern operating room equipped with a good air ventilation system and perhaps also "laminar flow" techniques, air exchange of several thousands of litres per hour may cause air currents that carry most of the oxygen away from the patient's airways. Figure 1 shows that very little of the oxygen reaches the alveoli in the first situation and that lowering the face mask has a dramatic

[1]Staff anesthesiologist, Department of Ophthalmology—Anesthesia, Helsinki University Central Hospital, SF-00290 Helsinki, Finland.

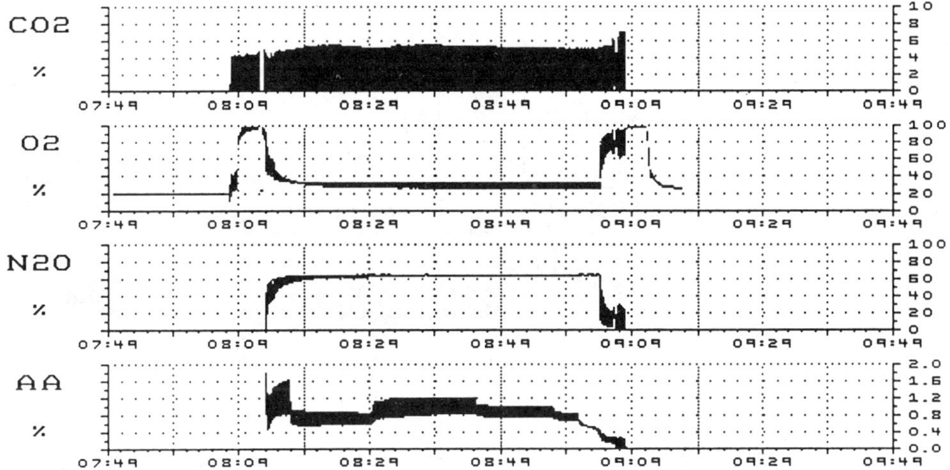

FIG. 1—*A trend of carbon dioxide (CO₂), oxygen (O₂), nitrous oxide (N₂O), and volatile anesthetic (AA, isoflurane) produced with a Capnomac multigas monitor and Daisy data acquisition system (Datex, Helsinki, Finland). The end-tidal oxygen concentration is initially relatively low when the face mask is held 5 cm above the face. Three minutes later it is lowered on the face. Isoflurane concentration changes are fairly rapid in this circle system with 3 L/min fresh gas flow.*

effect on alveolar oxygenation. After endotracheal intubation, inspiratory and expiratory oxygen concentrations are reversed due to nitrous oxide added into the circuit.

By using breath-by-breath oxygen and nitrous oxide monitoring, one could very rapidly achieve desired gas levels by adding high flows of nitrous oxide into the circuit for a short time. Rapid oxymetry enables monitoring of oxygen in both the circuit and mixed alveolar space. Simultaneous capnometry facilitates first confirmation of proper endotracheal intubation and thereafter the adjustment of sufficient alveolar ventilation to keep the carbon dioxide concentration at the desired level. The anesthetic agent tracing (AA, isoflurane) shows the initially large differences in the inspired and expired concentrations. Later, the vaporizer settings were adjusted in order to achieve the clinically desired alveolar concentrations in this patient. At the end of this anesthesia, the trends confirm safe emergence.

The quantitative administration of anesthetic agents aided by monitoring feedback can be applied to the use of vaporizers designed to release volatile anesthetic agents. The amount of anesthetic vapor entering the circuit is linearly dependent on the fresh gas minute flow which carries the agent into the circuit. The concentration dialed on the vaporizer may fairly accurately represent that in the fresh gas, but is thereafter diluted by the circuit volume and further diluted in the alveolar space. Figure 2 shows the relationships between the vaporizer dial and the inspired and end-tidal concentrations.

In nonrebreathing, high-flow techniques, changes in the inspired anesthetic gas concentration are reflected rapidly in the respective gas levels in the alveoli. Trends in Fig. 3 show rapidly stabilizing inspiratory and end-tidal concentrations of carbon dioxide, oxygen, nitrous oxide, and the anesthetic agent. End-tidal CO₂ is used to adjust the minute ventilation properly to yield normocapnia. The end-tidal oxygen level depends on the patient's oxygen consumption and fraction of inspired oxygen and is here adjusted to around 25%. That is approximately 10% above the normal. The same rapid changes in gas concentrations are seen at the end of this anesthetic where the patient starts to breathe spontaneously in response to increasing the CO₂ level after the vaporizer is turned off and the patient is extubated. Figure 4 gives a closer look at a high flow halogram. There is a slight delay before the

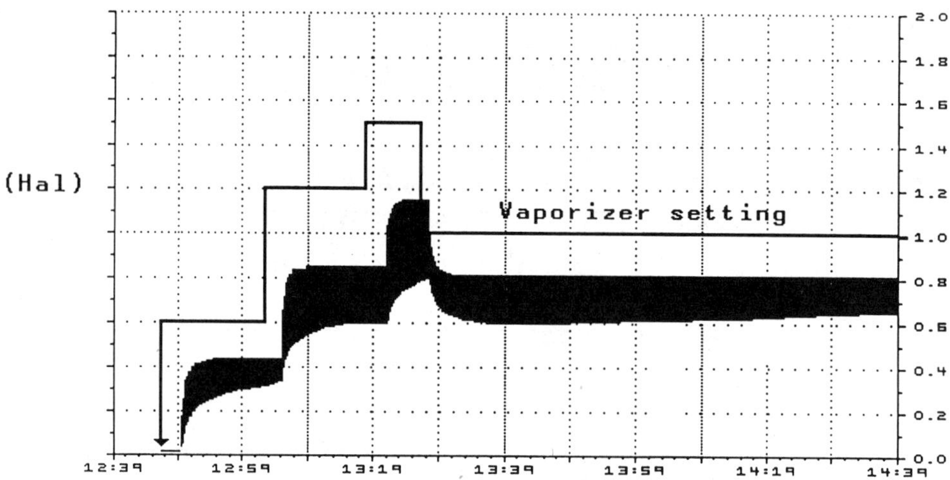

FIG. 2—*The relationships of the vaporizer setting and inspiratory and end-tidal halothane concentrations in a circle system with 3 L/min fresh gas flow. The envelope represents concentrations of the anesthetic agent inspired at the top and end-tidal at the bottom of the envelope. These concentrations are "reversed" after the vaporizer setting is abruptly decreased from 1.5 to 1% (at approximately 3:26 p.m.).*

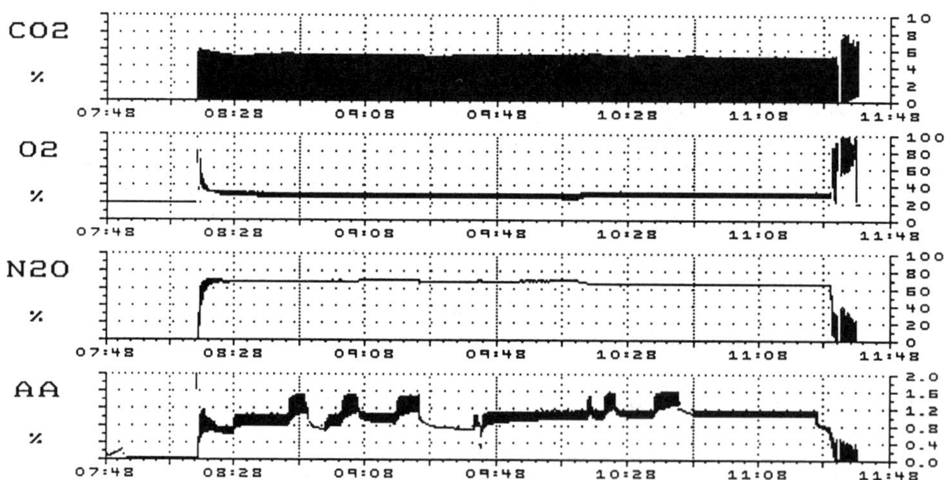

FIG. 3—*Comprehensive trends of the behavior of carbon dioxide (CO_2), oxygen (O_2), nitrous oxide (N_2O), and isoflurane (AA) in a nonrebreathing circuit.*

anesthetic agent reaches the Y-piece and the patient. Thereafter, the inspiratory concentration increases rapidly. Alveolar levels build up more slowly due to the buffering influence of the alveolar and lung tissue volumes and the pickup by pulmonary capillary perfusion. When the desired alveolar level is reached, the vaporizer is turned down. After an adjustment, 0.4% end-tidal is reached. Changes by 0.2% on the vaporized dial are followed by 0.1% changes in the end-tidal level. Turning off the vaporizer in a nonrebreathing circuit is rapidly reflected as near-zero inspiratory anesthetic agent concentrations. Note that at

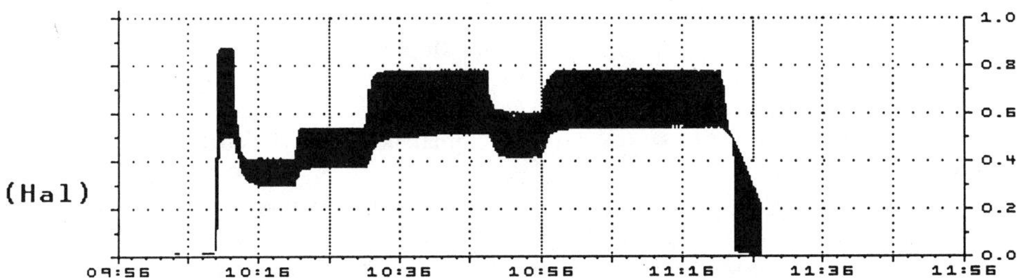

FIG. 4—*A closer look at a high flow halogram. Note the rapid initial increase in the end-tidal concentration and the ability to adjust the alveolar halothane levels with two-decimal accuracy.*

this point the inspired and end-tidal concentrations "turns over" (flips) and the end-tidal level falls rapidly.

The relationship between "end-tidal" and "alveolar" should be noted. Naturally, the end-tidal value is merely one observation during the respiratory cycle. The alveolar concentration fluctuates between maximal and minimal values generated by the effects of inspiratory gas concentration (enriching or diluting) and the movements of the specific gases along concentration gradients between the blood and the alveoli.

Reduction of the fresh gas flow in circle systems creates challenges in terms of oxygen and anesthetic agent supplies, and delayed response times to concentration changes. Most anesthesia ventilators are sensitive to changes in fresh gas minute flow. During every inspiration, the actual tidal volume is equal to the sum of the volume caused by the bellows and the volume of the fresh gas flowing into the system. Adjustments in the fresh gas flow will alter minute ventilation and necessitate adjustments of the tidal volume. Appropriate adjustments are most easily made by referring to the end-tidal carbon dioxide level. Figure 5 shows an initial increase in the end-tidal carbon dioxide concentration when fresh gas flow was reduced to 1.2 L/min. The oxygen trend aided in adjustments of proper gas mixture.

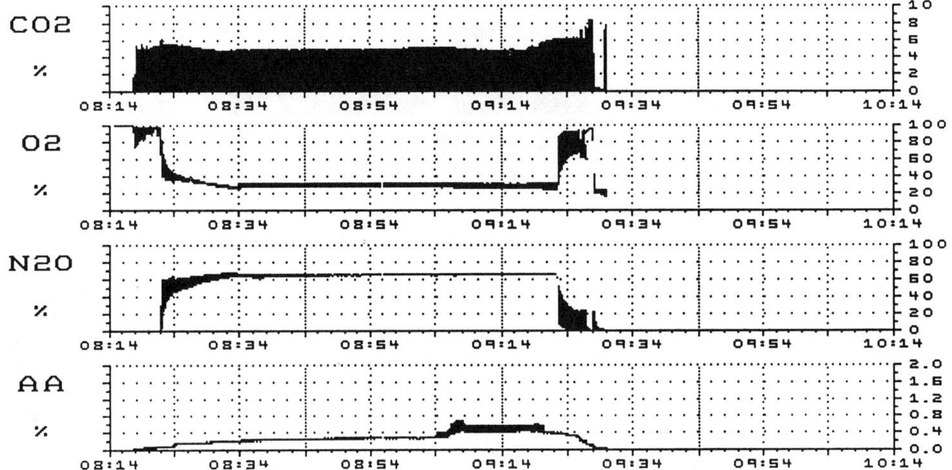

FIG. 5—*After endotracheal intubation, the fresh gas flow in a rebreathing circle system was lowered to 1.2 L/min. The vaporizer was set to 0.4%. Note the slow buildup of isoflurane concentration in the lungs.*

The trend of the corresponding anesthetic agent, in this case isoflurane, demonstrates the slow buildup of alveolar gas concentration when the dial was set to 0.4%. Such careful administration of potent inhalational anesthetics is often necessary in elderly patients. The combination of end-tidal oxygen and pulse oximetry allows for more accurate and safe adjustment of the fresh gas mixtures during minimal flow and closed use of rebreathing circuits.

The Mapleson D [3] or Bain [4] circuit is becoming increasingly popular. Due to the partial rebreathing, when used with fresh gas flows producing normal carbon dioxide tensions, the changes in alveolar anesthetic agent concentrations are very rapid. Figure 6 depicts the short alveolar gas level equilibration times following changes in inspired isoflurane concentrations. The vaporizer was turned off several times to demonstrate the rapid gas concentration changes when using this circuit. In this context it is necessary to point out that attempts to shorten induction times by high vaporizer dial settings may easily lead to an overdosage.

Temporarily high anesthetic agent concentrations may also be detected when anesthetic agents are injected directly into closed rebreathing circuits. Liquid injections could be made safer if continuous monitoring instead of rigid nonindividual dosage regimens were the basis of administration.

Volatile anesthetics depress the respiratory center in a dose-dependent manner. Before the advent of halometers it was common to anesthetize spontaneously breathing children so that their end-tidal CO_2 levels were between 7 to 7.5%, which normally could be reached by setting the vaporizer dial to 1.3 to 1.5% with 5-L fresh gas flow ($O_2:N_2O = 2:3$) in a Jackson-Rees circuit [5].

Monitoring in the recovery room is often based on miscellaneous equipment left over from the operating rooms. However, residual effects of anesthetics render patients vulnerable to complications arising out of initially relatively minor problems in the airways or depressed respiratory drive. Gas monitoring in the recovery room is hampered by sampling problems. The best solution in our experience has been to create a "preferred airway." A nasopharyngeal tube can easily be applied before the patient actually wakes up and can be used as an excellent sampling site for several hours, if necessary.

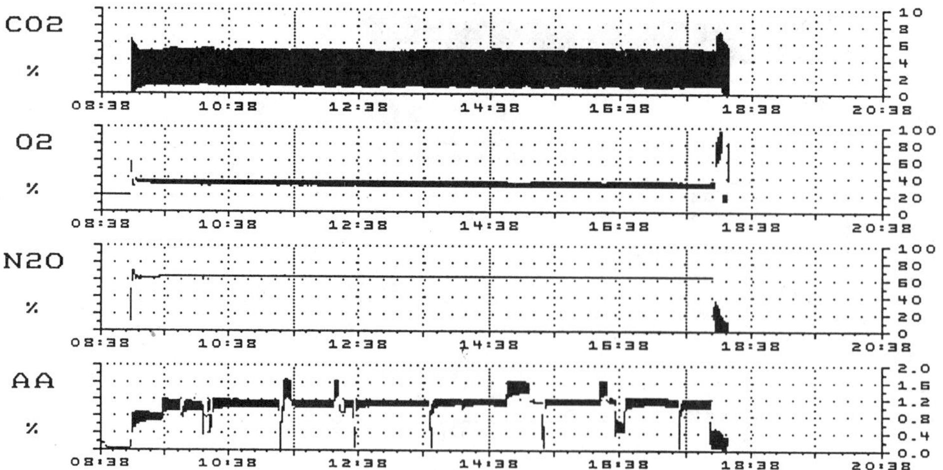

FIG. 6—*The vaporizer was turned off several times and on several times to demonstrate the rapid changes in isoflurane concentrations in a Mapleson D (Bain) [3] system. The three other gases remained very stable throughout the operation.*

Dozing, apneas, and low end-tidal oxygen and arterial saturation values are surprisingly common in the recovery room. In a small study on 44 patients breathing room air after 30 min of additional oxygen, we observed 19 patients with occasional desaturations below 85%. In all these patients, low end-tidal oxygen levels were noted 20 to 30 s prior to the low peripheral arterial blood saturation values. This suggests that monitoring principles in the recovery room should be reappraised.

The privilege to administer anesthesia is the practice of a risky business. The development of more comprehensive monitoring methods and equipment easily detracts us from physical contact with the patient. Although sensors and probes analyze factors we cannot otherwise sense, the dilemma is evident and needs to be solved. Quantitative analysis of both gases and halocarbon vapors is informative of gas delivery, uptake, and distribution [6,7], provides useful information on patient management, and enhances patient safety.

References

[1] Standard Specification for Minimum Performance and Safety Requirements for Components and Systems of Anesthesia Gas Machines, ASTM Standard F 1161-88, American Society for Testing and Materials, Philadelphia, 1989.

[2] Dorsch, J. A. and Dorsch, S. E., *Understanding Anesthesia Equipment*, 2nd ed., Williams and Wilkins, Baltimore, 1984.

[3] Mapleson, W. W., *British Journal of Anaesthesia*, Vol. 26, 1954, p. 323.

[4] Bain, J. A. and Spoerel, W. E., *Canadian Anaesthesia Society Journal*, Vol. 20, 1972, p. 426.

[5] Jackson-Rees, G., *British Medical Journal*, Vol. 2, 1950, p. 1419.

[6] Linko, K. and Paloheimo, M., *Critical Care Medicine*, Vol. 17, 1989, p. 345.

[7] Linko, K. and Paloheimo, M., *Journal of Clinical Monitoring*, Vol. 5, 1989, p. 149.

Michael J. Halsey[1]

Review of Methodology in Anesthetic Gas Monitoring

REFERENCE: Halsey, M. J., **"Review of Methodology in Anesthetic Gas Monitoring,"** *Continuous Anesthesia Gas Monitoring, ASTM STP 1090*, J. Hedley-Whyte and P. W. Thompson, Eds., American Society for Testing and Materials, Philadelphia, 1990, pp. 26–34.

ABSTRACT: This review concentrates on the underlying principles of operation of analyzers suitable for anesthetic gas monitoring. It includes any special advantage or disadvantage of a particular technique and relates these to the clinical requirements associated with patient safety. The methods available are categorized into those based on bulk properties, on spectroscopy, and on special applications such as mass spectrometry and gas chromatography. The final conclusion from the detailed considerations is that a performance standard for anesthesia gas monitoring is desirable and timely.

KEY WORDS: response times, spectroscopy, mass spectrometry, gas chromatography

There are many potential methods for the measurement of the gaseous concentrations of general anesthetics, and new approaches have recently been developed. This review does not attempt to be a comprehensive catalogue, but instead concentrates on the underlying principles of operation and indicates any special advantages or disadvantages of a technique. The most important context in which these instruments are used is during a surgical operation, and it is relevant to note that if the anesthetic monitor gives you the *wrong* answer, it will definitely compromise patient safety. That is not as trite a comment as it might seem because anesthetists for whom I have a great respect have a touching faith in impressive monitors. They believe the numbers. In the vast majority of cases they are right. But the sad fact is that there are a number of factors that mean the answers may be inaccurate or inappropriate. So recognition of the performance limitations of any instrument is a critical issue.

Performance limitations have to be matched against the clinical requirements, and the latter divide into two broad types: (*a*) analyses of discrete samples of a gas assumed to have a homogeneous composition, such as that from the input or output of an anesthetic machine; (*b*) on-line analysis of a variable gas flow of varying composition such as that from the expired air of a patient. Inevitably these two broad categories do not fit all the requirements. For example, monitoring of anesthetic gases in the general atmosphere of an operating room uses a representative sample that includes variations in composition dependent on both time and location.

These different types of clinical requirements for gas monitoring lead to the identification of the important performance characteristics which apply to all methods. These include speed of response, specificity, and selectivity. The first of these will be considered separately; the other two will be included in the discussions of the alternative methodologies.

[1]Head of High Pressure Neurological Syndrome Research Group, Division of Anaesthesia, Clinical Research Centre, Harrow, Middlesex, United Kingdom.

Response Time

Knowledge of the response times of gas analyzers is essential when rapidly changing gas concentrations are being studied. The measurements are not accurate if the instrument does not respond rapidly enough for its output to reach the actual concentration at the end of each breath. This problem has been widely recognized [1], but there is still much confusion over the different methods of specifying response times, over the different factors altering response times, and over the relationship between inadequate response time and inaccurate concentration measurements.

Figure 1 illustrates some of the different terms used in specifying response times. In addition to the terms used in the figure, the "rise time" can also be defined as the time taken for the output to respond to a sudden step change in concentration. This response can be either for the output changing from 10% of the final value to 90% of the final value (T_{90}) or from 10 to 70% of the final value (T_{70}). Both definitions avoid assumptions about the reproducibility of the precise changes of the response curves outside these limits.

The problems come not with these formal definitions but with the practical interpretation

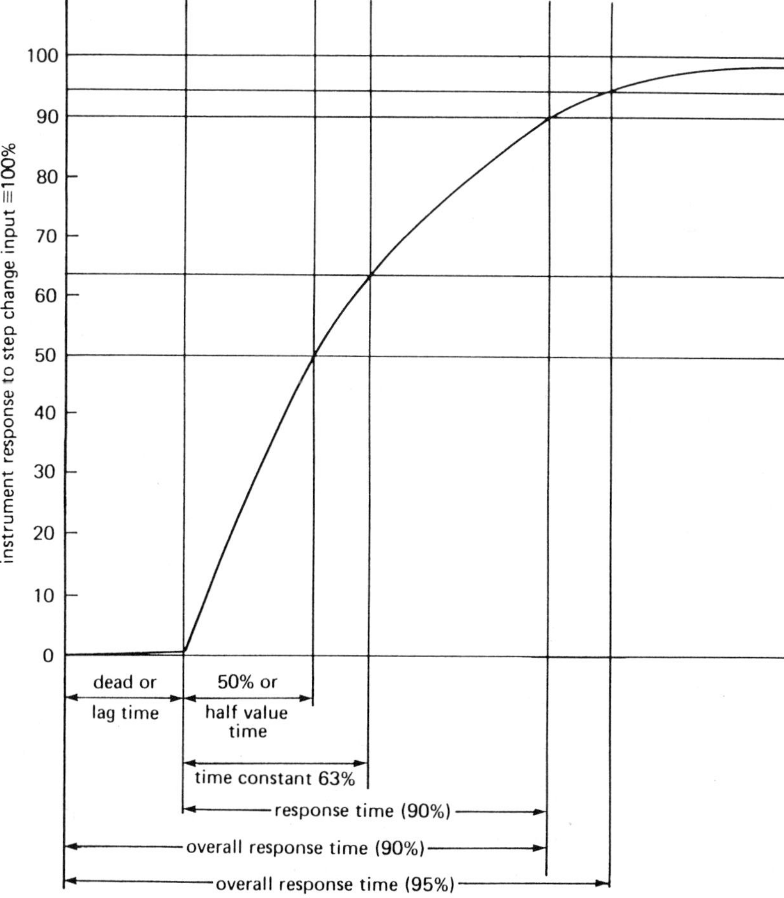

FIG. 1—*Definitions of various terms used in the description of response times.*

of these definitions. When a standard is written, the equipment is compared by many authorities with the specifications in the standard. The response time of the equipment must be written in a form which will allow evaluation. That includes evaluation of the accompanying material that the manufacturer has to provide.

It appears that some manufacturers are failing to provide the necessary information on response times, and that many are stating response times which are grossly misleading. The authorities must always be sophisticated enough to pick this up.

Experience with U.S. manufacturers of gas analyzers indicates that they specify a response time and almost universally confuse that with rise time. Part of the reason is that the engineering definition is very much what you put up, but the practical definition from the point of view of deciding what respiratory rate you can follow is really rise time and not lag time. However, many manufacturers now specify a lag time with a certain configuration and sample flow rate or, in the case of mainstream or nondiverting devices, an airway adapter dead space and separately list the rise time—almost universally with the parentheses 10–90%.

The electronic rise time issue must be distinguished from the pneumatics. For example, one factor is the profound effect of putting any kind of filter on the analyzer. In many cases it seems necessary. Some manufacturers have produced analyzers and then subsequently said it is necessary to put a filter on to prevent it getting bunged up with mucus. That may double or even treble the response time; this is all unstated.

The importance of knowing the response times is that they give some indication whether, at a given respiratory rate, the analyzer can "see" the end-tidal concentration. Unfortunately the position is further complicated because the response time on its own is not enough. You also have to specify or make some assumption about the shape of the respiratory waveform. If we are talking about end-tidal concentrations, the part of the waveform we are interested in is the expiratory time. So it is very hard to make generalizations. However, the overall conclusion from this subsection is that a long rise time will result in a systematic error in one direction and not a noise error, which many clinicians incorrectly assume it is.

Classifications of Gas Analysis

The methods currently available divide into chemical and physicochemical. The latter group are more important for the anesthetic gases and further subdivide into three categories: (1) those based on bulk properties, e.g., refractive index and thermal conductivity; (2) those utilizing one of several varieties of spectroscopy; and (3) the so-called specific methods, which include gas chromatography and mass spectrometry. The classification for a particular method is not always obvious because the fundamental mode of detection is complicated by a secondary method of transduction. For example, one of the piezoelectric anesthetic gas monitors is in fact a simple nonspecific bulk property detector measuring the perturbation of the mass of the detector following absorption of the anesthetic.

Chemical Methods

The chemical methods of gas analysis are usually thought of as being primarily for oxygen or carbon dioxide and are associated with Haldane and Scholander apparatus. The principle of operation is differential absorption, and although they are slow and suitable for discrete samples only, they have the advantage of being accurate and providing a primary standard for use in calibration of either instrument. The accuracy is of the order of $\pm 0.05\%$ of the total sample. Theoretically, it should be possible to develop similar chemical methods for the volatile and gaseous anesthetics, but this has not yet been achieved satisfactorily.

Physical Methods Based on Bulk Properties

These methods are nonspecific and include density balance, refractometry, and thermal conductivity. Of these methods, refractometry is still widely used in the calibration of outputs from anesthetic vaporizers and has been thought, incorrectly, to be an absolute method. Its use requires a knowledge of the refractive index of the particular anesthetic being measured, and this, in turn, requires a knowledge of the anesthetic concentrations. Thus, as with most other methods of analysis, it is comparative rather than absolute. The considerations of the preparation of absolute standards are outside the scope of this review, but there are a surprising number of factors to be considered and the resulting calibration mixtures are not always satisfactory.

One additional method in the category of bulk properties is absorption into either an elastomer or a film coating on a vibrating crystal. The absorption causes the matrix to expand, to increase in mass, and to change its elastic properties. These perturbations can be sensed in a variety of ways. One of the most interesting aspects of this method of measurement is that the molecular changes in elastomers produced by anesthetics may resemble one component of the changes taking place at the biological sites of action of general anesthetics. This implies that it may be possible to construct an instrument capable of measuring anesthetic potencies rather than just anesthetic concentrations (i.e., a MAC meter). In addition, the methodology would apply to either a gaseous or a liquid medium [2].

Spectroscopy

Compounds absorb and subsequently emit energy that is a characteristic both of the compound and of its concentration. The usual methods of spectroscopy rely on the fact that each anesthetic absorbs energy at a particular wave length or group of wavelengths. For convenience, the spectrum of wavelength is usually divided into regions: ultraviolet (200 to 400 nm), visible (380 to 750 nm), and infrared (1 to 15 μm). The anesthetic gases do not absorb light in the visible region of the spectrum and are therefore colorless (in the gas phase but not in the liquid where preservatives such as thymol have been added). Figure 2 illustrates the ranges of the different wavelengths, and it should not be forgotten that these include those used in nuclear magnetic resonance, which has a future potential for measuring anesthetic concentrations in tissues and blood but probably will not be suitable for gas measurements.

The absorption of energy by a compound is described by quantum theory, and high resolution spectroscopy reveals the more detailed spectra underneath broad absorption bands

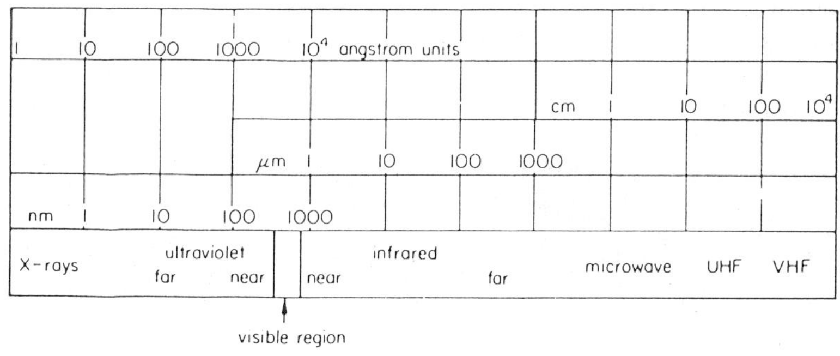

FIG. 2—*Wavelengths of various radiations used in different types of spectroscopy.*

(Fig. 3). Theoretically these could provide the basis for a more sophisticated agent specific analyzer.

Commonly, analyzers cover the infrared region, where most gases absorb energy. The exceptions are the simple nonpolar diatomic gases such as oxygen and nitrogen. The method does have some degree of selectivity because different anesthetics absorb at different wavelengths within the region, and it is possible to differentiate between, say, carbon dioxide and nitrous oxide by selecting the appropriate wavelength. However, it is more difficult to differentiate between halothane and nitrous oxide, for example, since both absorb in similar regions of the infrared spectrum. Fortunately, halothane also absorbs energy in the ultraviolet region, where it is unaffected by other anesthetic agents.

Another interfering component of all anesthetic gas samples is water. In some instances attempts have been made to remove it before analysis; in others deliberate wavelength ranges are selected to avoid the problem (Fig. 4). An alternative approach is the use of different wavelength ranges for detector and source as well as using the windows of the sample cell as a wavelength filter (Fig. 5).

Apart from the simple error of one absorption band of a gas overlapping another, there is the so-called pressure or collision-broadening effect. When a particular gas absorbs energy it becomes energized, and the energized molecule then can collide with a molecule of a different gas and give up its energy. Thus, another component of the gas mixture may take up energy indirectly by "collision broadening," although it does not itself absorb energy directly at the selected wavelength. The error is particularly notorious in carbon dioxide measurements when nitrogen, nitrous oxide, or cyclopropane are present in the sample but not in the calibrating gas.

In general, all absorption methods have an output which is nonlinear with respect to changes in concentration. This is because the equation for the absorption of energy by a sample has a logarithmic form (Beer-Lambert laws). This has led manufacturers to use microprocessors to linearize the curve (Fig. 6). The difficulty with this approach is that the shape of the overall curve may be changed by environmental factors, and what is suitable in the laboratory fails when used in the operating room.

A recent development in anesthetic gas monitors is an instrument based on Raman spectroscopy. When a beam of light passes through a medium a certain amount is absorbed, a certain amount transmitted, and a certain amount scattered. Some of the scattered light has its frequency or wavelength shifted because the collision has resulted in the loss of energy to the molecule. The intensity of Raman scattered light at specific frequencies gives an absolute measure of each gas concentration. The peaks for the physiological and anesthetic gases are separated from each other, and there is no cross sensitivity with water vapor, for example. The sample gases are not degraded by Raman scattering and can therefore be returned to the breathing system. Calibration requirements are simplified because the relative sensitivity to various gases is fixed, and so after an initial calibration for each gas, periodic recalibration against nitrogen and oxygen in room air is sufficient. The development

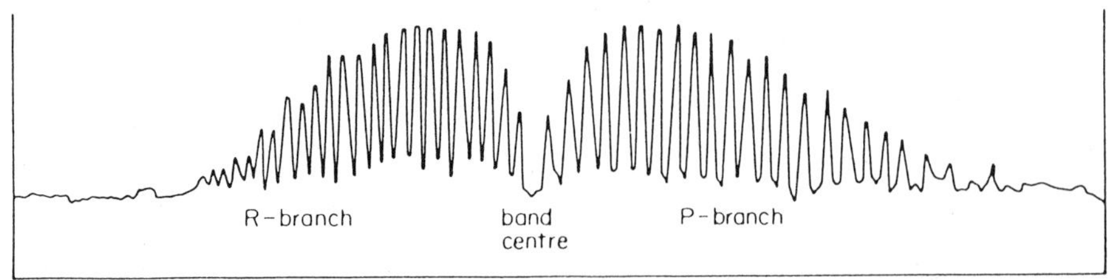

FIG. 3—*A high-resolution spectrum showing fine structure underlying the overall band.*

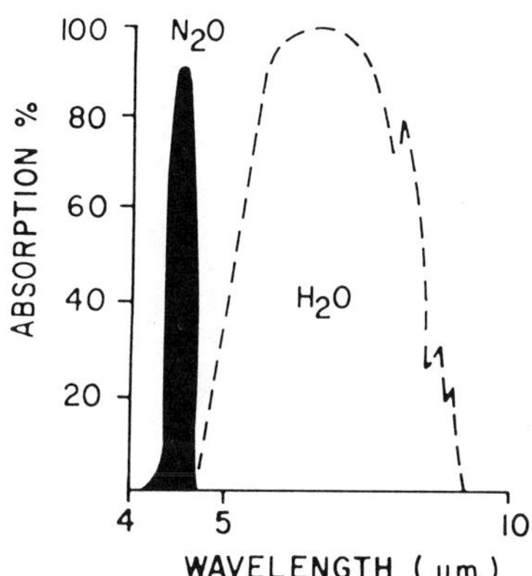

FIG. 4—*The infrared spectra of nitrous oxide and water vapor (courtesy of Hewlett-Packard Corp., Waltham, Massachusetts).*

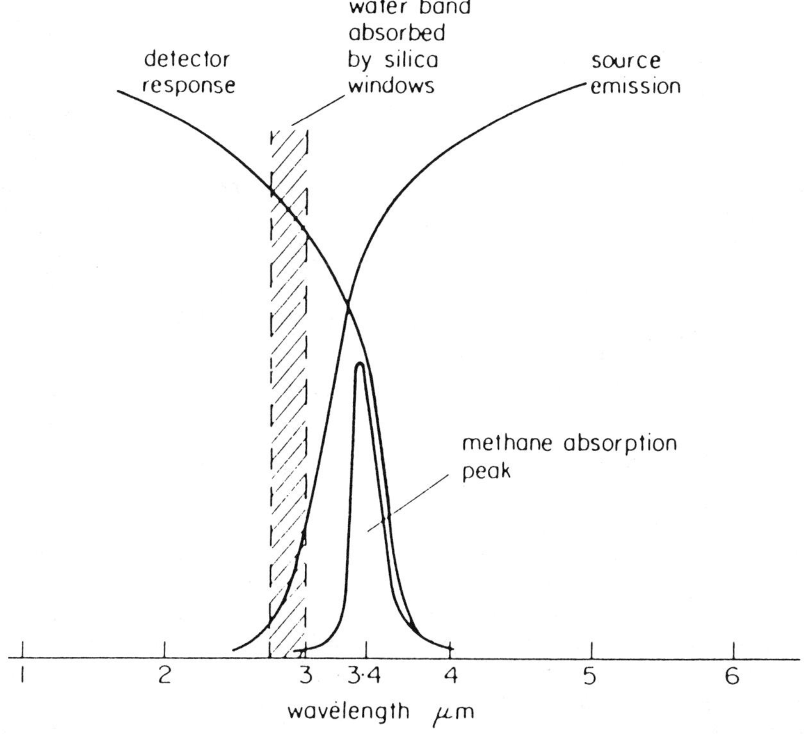

FIG. 5—*A simple selective source analyzer showing the overlap of source and detector responses (courtesy of Analysis Automation Ltd. Oxford).*

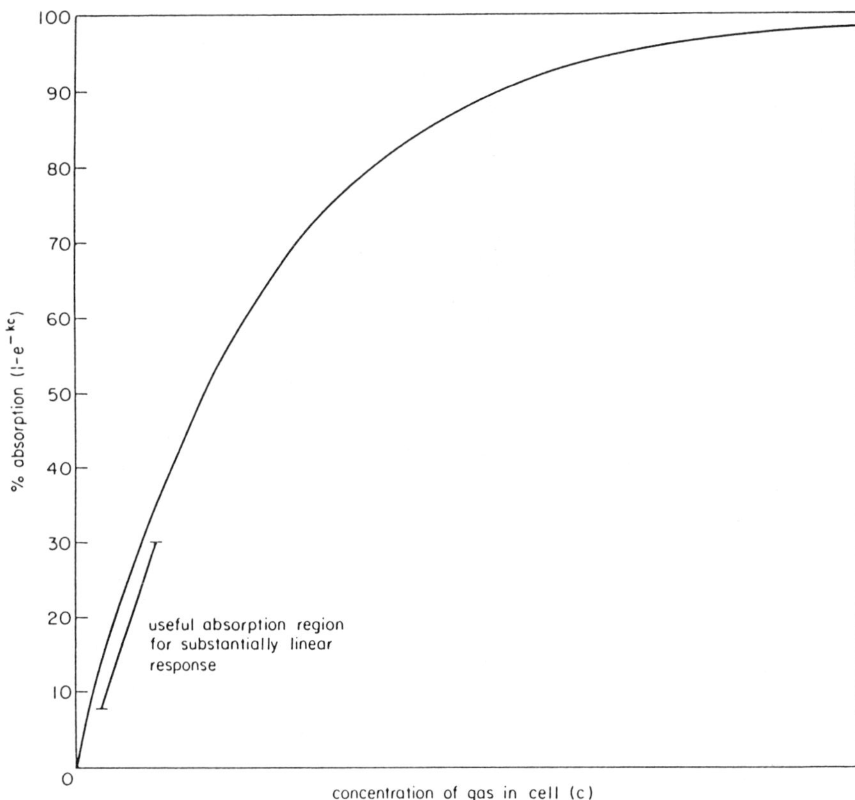

FIG. 6—*Optical absorption showing the nonlinear response associated with Beer's Law (courtesy of Analysis Automatic Ltd. Oxford).*

of small argon lasers as the light source has allowed the principles of Raman spectroscopy to be incorporated into a fast-responding dedicated multiple gas monitor which may provide an attractive alternative to the mass spectrometer [3,4].

Gas Chromatography and Mass Spectrometry

These physical techniques are established and well described [5], and only an outline of their principles will be included here.

The gas chromatograph first separates the components of a gas mixture and then measures their individual concentrations. The two most common detectors for anesthetic gases are the flame ionization detector, which is used for most organic gases, and the katharometer for inorganic gases. The method really is satisfactory only for discrete samples, but with suitable modification it can measure gas concentrations down to the parts-per-million range with the same percentage accuracy as at normal clinical concentrations. It is used for analyzing blood samples containing anesthetics as well as gas samples. It is also applicable to other drugs, and in one or other of its different forms (e.g., high pressure liquid chromatography) the basic methods will be found in every analytical laboratory.

The mass spectrometer separates components on the basis of their mass rather than by their chemical or physical properties. It is the mass/charge ratios of a component or its breakdown products which separate it in a magnetic field [6], but it is only now that truly reliable instruments which are easy to operate are coming into anesthesia research. One of the problems was that the technique was almost too versatile, and there were too many alternative methods of operation for the instrument to be used outside a specialized laboratory. However, such problems have now been overcome, and both size and cost have been reduced. The adaptation of the quadrupole mass spectrometer to multipatient anesthesia gas monitoring is being evaluated in several centers. It is necessary to have a pressure-stabilized long capillary inlet system and computer control of the quadrupole filter with timing, calibration, and subsequent analysis and display of the information for each operating room. At the moment there still appears to be problems with the signal-to-noise ratio when used with the multi-inputs, which particularly show up in the reproducibility and accuracy of the carbon dioxide measurements [7]. There is also some evidence of a rapid aging of the electron multipliers, probably because of the use of high concentrations of oxygen.

The use of long sampling tubes for remote patient monitoring by mass spectrometry has now been investigated both theoretically and experimentally. Mathematical models have been developed which predict the ideal geometry and material to minimize signal distortion and signal transmission delay. There are a limited number of commercially available tubes of the ideal radii for given lengths, and account also needs to be taken of gas-tube interactions. One solution proposed is a tube with an exponentially rising radius as a function of distance, rather than a uniform tube [8].

One of the initial problems with a mass spectrometer was that different gases might have the same mass peaks either from the parent compound or the breakdown products. The obvious example was carbon dioxide and nitrous oxide, which both have masses of 44 mass units. This was fairly easy to overcome because their breakdown products have different mass numbers. A more serious problem is when the components of the gas mixture are unknown. An example of this in anesthesia was the discovery that isoflurane partial pressures were being incorrectly measured with a mass spectrometer because fluorinated hydrocarbon propellants were in the air sample. Some fluorinated hydrocarbons generate a signal at mass 91, which is also the position for a strong isoflurane mass peak. At the time this mass spectrum overlap was unknown to the investigator, who incorrectly interpreted the signal as reflecting a high isoflurane concentration [9].

Conclusion

The writing of a standard for anesthetic gas monitoring is much needed and very important. It will be very difficult because of the differences in performance requirements and problems such as interfacing of equipment. However, the recognition of the complexities of the clinical requirements and the performance limitations of specific methodologies should make the task less formidable.

References

[1] Brunner, J. X. and Westenskow, D. R., *British Journal of Anaesthesia*, Vol. 61, 1988, pp. 628–638.

[2] White, D. C., Wardley-Smith, B., and Halsey, M. J., *British Journal of Anaesthesia*, Vol. 44, 1972, pp. 1020–1024.

[3] Van Wagenen, R. A., Westenskow, D. R., Berner, R. E., Gregoris, D. E., and Coleman, D. L., *Journal of Clinical Monitoring*, Vol. 2, 1986, pp. 215–222.

[4] Westenskow, D. R., Coleman, D. L., Gregoris, D. E., Smith, K. W., and Van Wagenen, R. A., *Journal of Clinical Monitoring*, Vol. 3, 1987, pp. 1020–1024.

[5] Sykes, M. K., Vickers, M. D., and Hull, C. J., *Principles of Clinical Measurement*, Blackwell, Oxford, 1981.

[6] Fowler, K. T., *Physics of Medicine and Biology*, Vol. 14, 1969, pp. 185–199.
[7] Salamonsen, R. F., Tulloh, A. H., and Boyd, T., *Anaesthesia and Intensive Care*, Vol. 14, 1986, pp. 163–173.
[8] Lerou, J. G. C., Von Egmond, J., and Kalmer, B. H. H., *Clinical Physics and Physiological Measurement*, Vol. 7, 1986, pp. 125–137.
[9] Gravenstein, N., Theisen, G. J., and Knudsen, A. K., *Anesthesiology*, Vol. 62, 1985, pp. 70–72.

Brian D. Joyner[1]

Is There an Anesthetic Contribution to Ozone Depletion or Greenhouse Warming?

REFERENCE: Joyner, B. D., **"Is There an Anesthetic Contribution to Ozone Depletion or Greenhouse Warming?"** *Continuous Anesthesia Gas Monitoring, ASTM STP 1090,* J. Hedley-Whyte and P. W. Thompson, Eds., American Society for Testing and Materials, Philadelphia, 1990, pp. 35–46.

ABSTRACT: Chlorofluorocarbons (CFCs) are firmly linked with stratospheric ozone depletion and potential global atmospheric warming—the greenhouse effect. Halogenated anesthetics—halothane, enflurane, and isoflurane—are superficially similar in chemical structure to CFCs, and concern has been expressed regarding their possible contribution to the same environmental issues.

The historical development of both concerns is traced, together with the chemical structures of the highly stable CFCs and of the less stable substitute materials now under development. From this information it is shown that any conceivable contribution to either issue by halogenated anesthetics would be absolutely minimal.

On a production volume basis alone, the annual world production of anesthetics is about one thousand times less than that of CFCs. In addition, the chemical structures of anesthetics show much more similarity with the "environment-friendly" substitutes for CFCs than with CFCs.

KEY WORDS: halogenated anesthetics, chlorofluorocarbons, ozone depletion, global warming

Chlorofluorocarbons (CFCs) are implicated in stratospheric ozone depletion and also play a part in absorption of radiation from the earth's surface, contributing to the greenhouse warming effect. Recognition of the superficial chemical similarity between halogenated anesthetics and CFCs has led to suggestions that these gases are also implicated. Improving standards of control of anesthetic gases and reducing concentrations in the general atmosphere of the operating theatre are usually achieved by venting waste gases to the atmosphere, so there is no doubt that anesthetics are released.

Depletion of stratospheric ozone could lead to increased levels of damaging ultraviolet radiation (UV-B) reaching the earth. The greenhouse warming of the atmosphere could result in major climate changes and extensive flooding of low-lying areas as sea levels rise. It is significant to note that the difference in global average temperature between an ice age and the present temperate climate is only around 4°C.

I will discuss CFCs and why we have them. Let's go back to the 1920s when refrigeration depended on ammonia, sulphur dioxide, or methyl chloride—all flammable, poisonous, or noxious. The United States was getting ready for domestic refrigeration, but nobody wanted those sorts of refrigerants in their kitchens. Frigidaire, a division of General Motors, in 1928 commissioned a bright chemist called Thomas Midgley to come up with a safe chemical that had the same physical properties, i.e., that produced the same refrigerating effect. In a matter of weeks he devised chlorofluorocarbons (CFCs). Domestic refrigeration took off from there, with the ubiquitous name of "Freon," though that is Dupont's trademark.

[1]Business development manager, ISC Chemicals Ltd, Avonmouth, Bristol BS11 9YF.

Chemically, CFCs are compounds that contain nothing but carbon, chlorine, and fluorine (Fig. 1). Of the three structures, the top two—trichlorofluoromethane and dichlorodifluoromethane—are the most common. There is also an ethane series. The names are extremely similar, making it easy to make a typing error, so the industry worldwide has adopted the numbering system, 11, 12, 113, and so on.

The properties of CFCs are such that they have the right physical characteristics to do the job. They have very high levels of chemical stability and compatibility with materials of construction. They are nonflammable, virtually nontoxic, and odorless. They are ideal for most applications to which they are put, but the high level of chemical compatibility leads us into the theory of ozone depletion.

These fully halogenated materials build up in the troposphere and slowly migrate to the stratosphere—slowly because 90% of the atmosphere is actually in the troposphere (that is, up to 10 to 12 km altitude) and only 10% is in the stratosphere. There is roughly a 10% interchange every year. As a first approximation, something emitted at ground level takes ten years to get to the stratosphere.

Photodecomposition in the stratosphere releases chlorine. Chlorine catalytically converts ozone to molecular oxygen and chlorine oxide. This means less ozone, which has the role of filtering out high-level UV radiation. Therefore, there could be an increase in UV radiation at ground level, which could lead to the effects mentioned.

A brief timetable: in 1972, before the hypothesis first surfaced, the CFC industry realized that all uses for these compounds meant that sooner or later they were released to the atmosphere. This was most obvious with aerosol propellants and most delayed with their use in refrigeration or thermal insulating foam, where the compounds can be locked up for many years. And so we commissioned scientific studies to see what the effects of CFCs would be in the atmosphere. One of these programs measured air samples.

The first findings showed that CFCs were present in significant levels and were increasing. That led Rowland and Molina [1] in 1974 to formulate their hypothesis of ozone depletion. In 1978 the U.S. Environmental Protection Agency (EPA) restricted use of CFCs in aerosols, but not other uses. In 1980, the European Economic Community (EEC) adopted a measure to freeze production capacity and asked the aerosol industry to implement a voluntary reduction of 30%, which it did.

In 1985 the United Nations Environment Programme (UNEP) finalized the Vienna Convention for the protection of the ozone layer, but without specifying any particular compounds. In 1987 came the Montreal Protocol, a rider to the convention, dealing with CFCs and also the halon bromofluorocarbons, gases which are rather different. On 1 Jan. 1989, the Protocol entered into force, having been signed by 30 or 35 countries representing more than 85% of world production and use of CFCs. But a few crucial countries were omitted.

Global ozone varies enormously from time to time, season to season, and from one part of the world to another. The global average is about 300 Dobson units—an arbitrary measure: Dobson devised a spectrophotometer technique for measuring ozone in the atmosphere, and the unit is named after him. On a global average over the last 20 or so years, ozone

Chlorofluorocarbons

CCl_3F	trichlorofluoromethane	CFC 11
CCl_2F_2	dichlorodifluoromethane	CFC 12
CCl_2FCClF_2	trichlorotrifluoroethane	CFC 113

FIG. 1—*Chlorofluorocarbons.*

has stayed within $\pm 3\%$—but that smooths out all the local seasonal and regional variations, which are very considerable.

Figure 2 is a depiction of the Antarctic ozone depletion or "hole" on one day in October 1986. It is clear that there is a very substantial loss of ozone at 12 to 24 km altitude, with very little difference at lower or higher altitudes. The reason for the term "hole" is that when computer-generated ozone density maps are produced from satellite data, and a dark color is chosen for the area of lowest ozone, the resulting picture looks like a hole. It is not as if all the ozone had disappeared from the atmosphere above Antarctica, but it had been substantially reduced. This effect was discovered to be happening each austral spring, starting mid-September and running into November. Why?

The reason is the peculiar weather conditions that pertain during the Antarctic night, aided by the circumpolar winds. Antarctica is an island with enormous areas of ocean around it. There is a steady wind pattern round and round Antarctica—the so-called Roaring Forties—which produces an inner vortex of air which is essentially contained by these circular winds. During the Antarctic night, the temperature drops to below minus 80°C, cold enough for polar stratospheric clouds to form. These are initially ice particles but gradually become clouds of nitric acid particles as nitrogen oxides freeze out on the surface of the ice. You have in a sense a chemical containment vessel, the walls of which are the winds circulating around Antarctica. As the sun comes back in the spring, there is a peculiar chemistry within the vortex, leading to ozone depletion. As the vortex breaks up and the atmosphere warms, levels return to normal, but this does not happen the same way every year.

Now we come to the 1987 campaign. An expedition mounted by NASA and supported by many scientists from around the world, including the UK Meteorological Office, flew two aircraft from the southernmost tip of South America (Punta Arenas in Chile). One was the ER2, the modern scientific version of the U2 spy plane, which flies at about 18 to 22 km altitude, i.e., in the stratosphere, but has limited range and can carry only automatic equipment. The other was a DC8 carrying about 40 scientists with all their equipment, a

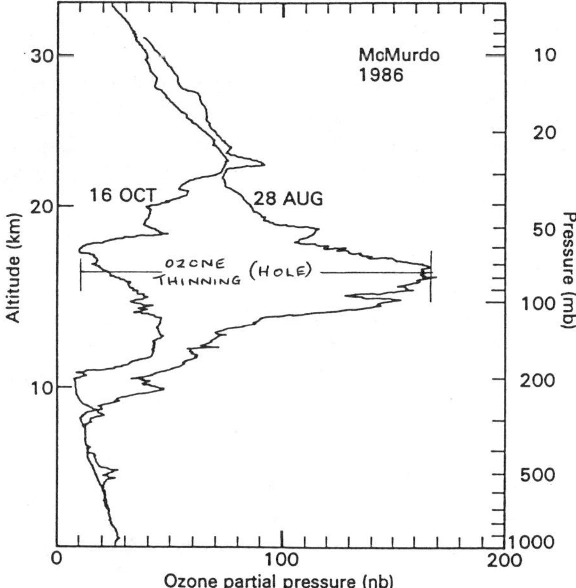

FIG. 2—*Ozone profiles from balloon soundings over McMurdo Station, Antarctica.*

real flying laboratory. The DC8 flies at 10 to 12 km. The two together give the opportunity to make measurements at different levels in the atmosphere and are supplemented by balloon and ground-based instruments from the various permanent bases in Antarctica such as Halley Bay, McMurdo, and Amundsen-Scott base at the pole itself.

In 1987 the overall picture was one of very substantial levels of ozone depletion. In 1988 there were no flights, but all the ground-based and satellite measurements were made, and the ozone hole was a virtual nonevent. Ozone dropped by 50%, and that decrease lasted for 60 to 70 days in 1987; in 1988 it dropped by 15% and lasted 12 days, which is an indication of the variation that can occur.

A similar campaign in the Arctic ran from 1 Jan. to 14 Feb. 1989. The same two aircraft, flying out of Stavanger in Norway and supplemented by balloon and ground-based measurements made in the Shetlands, Greenland, Northern Canada, and Russia, found that the same basic chemistry conditions are there, i.e., polar stratospheric clouds with high levels of chlorine oxides and low levels of nitrogen oxides. But there is no ozone depletion. That is not surprising because the sun has not yet reached the high Arctic and there is only a small polar vortex. Whether the vortex will still be there containing the conditions for unusual chemistry when the sun gets to the high Arctic is impossible to predict.

What it comes down to is chlorine in the atmosphere. There is a background level of chlorine which comes from volcanic eruptions and from sea spray, and also methyl chloride, the vast majority of which comes from the sea. And then there are man-made chlorocarbon compounds, methyl chloroform and carbon tetrachloride being two notable ones, and finally there are CFCs. So there is a background, mostly natural with man-made additions, and then that part due to CFCs. As the level of chlorine rises in the atmosphere, so the predictions of eventual larger scale ozone depletion are supported.

Figure 3 is the sort of chemistry that was always understood as happening in the atmosphere when Dobson first started measuring ozone [2]. High-energy UV radiation broke down oxygen molecules into atoms, and atoms could recombine into ozone. Ozone in turn was broken down by the same high-energy radiation, and this was the filtering mechanism that absorbed high-energy UV radiation to reform oxygen molecules and atoms. It was quickly realized that this was not enough to account for the ozone balance in the atmosphere and that there must be something else. In turn, water vapor, nitrogen oxides, and finally chlorine became implicated.

When we come to the peculiar conditions that obtain in the Antarctic and possibly the Arctic, unusual compounds are formed. Normally, chlorine interacts with ozone to give chlorine oxide and oxygen. Chlorine oxide can combine with nitrogen dioxide to form chlorine nitrate: this is a sink, a stable compound which will eventually be rained out of the atmosphere. Similarly, chlorine oxide can combine with water vapor to form hydrogen chloride (hydrochloric acid). That also can be washed out of the atmosphere. So these, in the normal atmosphere, are methods by which active chlorine is removed and thus cannot interfere with ozone.

At temperatures below $-80°C$, those compounds combine on the surface of ice crystals

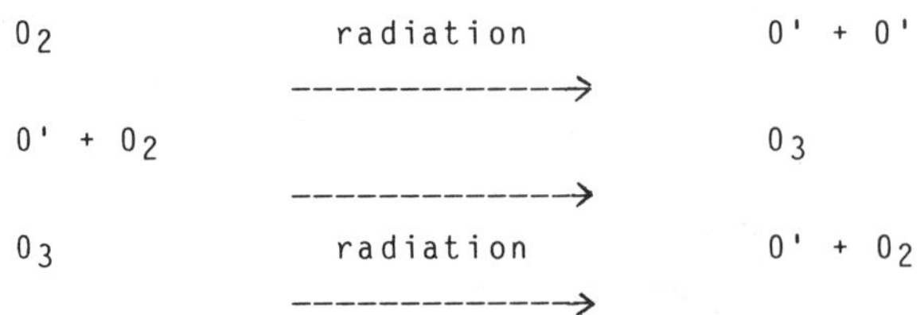

FIG. 3—*Reactions of oxygen important in Antarctic ozone formation.*

in the atmosphere to give nitric acid, which is dissolved and produces polar stratospheric clouds of nitric acid and releases chlorine. The chlorine can be broken down by UV radiation to form chlorine atoms, and so the cycle goes on. This is basically what happens in the Antarctic as the sun comes back at the end of the polar night. This highly unusual, perturbed chemistry takes place releasing ample chlorine to decompose ozone. Measurements in the atmosphere show high levels of chlorine oxides with low levels of ozone. By sampling and analyzing the polar stratospheric clouds, it was determined that they are made of nitric acid.

There has also been a major review of ozone measurement data on a global basis, from which some trends have been deduced. From 1969–86, at certain latitude bands in the northern hemisphere and at certain times of the year, there are statistically significant reductions in column ozone concentrations. This is most apparent in winter between 50 and 60° North, with lesser effects in the 30 to 40° and 40 to 50° bands.

The precise ozone values are open to debate and certainly vary with the statistical treatment of the data, but it now seems clear that this is an actual effect. But we must remember that one problem with measuring ozone from ground-based instruments is that in large parts of the world you can have no ground-based instruments because there is no land. So ground-based coverage is very patchy. Measurement stations are concentrated in the USA and Western Europe, with some in Russia, one or two in China, India, and so on. Because there is not a lot of land in the southern hemisphere, the sites are concentrated in the north. So to talk of a global average ozone measurement is difficult.

However, assume that the trend is correct, that there is a real ozone depletion of a few percent over the last 15 years. Figure 4 shows plots of actual UV irradiation at a variety of stations in the USA, ranging from El Paso in Texas or Albuquerque in New Mexico up to Minneapolis. That is, they cover the same latitude bands as the indicated ozone depletion. Those lines head downwards: there was less UV irradiation when there should have been more. Other factors such as increasing air pollution may be involved, so all that this em-

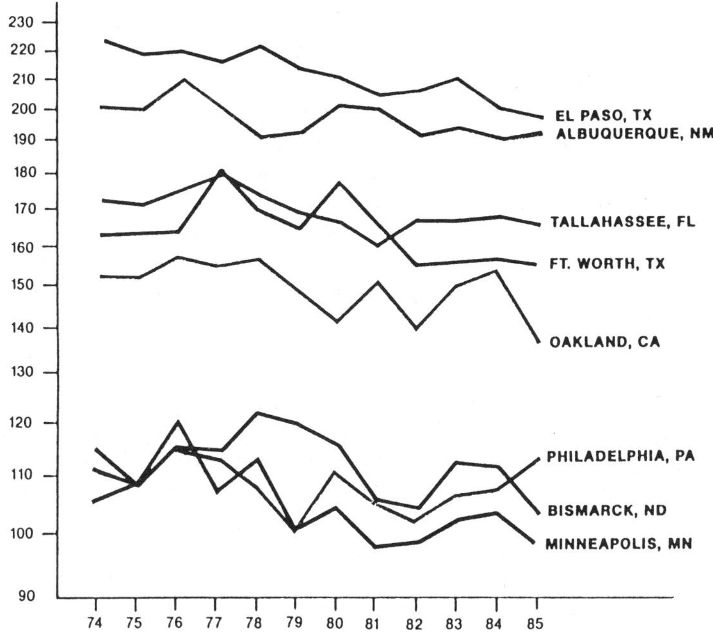

FIG. 4—*UV irradiance levels (from Scotto et al. [5]).*

phasizes is that the science is far from clearcut. A recent paper [3] has indicated that a 10% increase in cloud cover, a possible consequence of greenhouse warming, could more than swamp the increase in UV radiation from a likely ozone decrease. So greenhouse warming and ozone depletion are very clearly linked together in their eventual effects.

In the Montreal Protocol, 1986 is the baseline for statistical data. The Protocol came into force at the beginning of 1989. From the middle of 1989 there will be a freeze on production and use of CFCs. My company has already given a commitment to the UK government, which is acting on behalf of the European Community in this case, that we will not produce and sell from July 1989 onwards more per year than we did in 1986. And come the middle of 1993, we will cut back by at least 20% and by 1998 by at least 50%. All of the western CFC-producing countries are parties to this Protocol. The countries that are not part of it at the moment are Russia, China, India, and many others. This is the reason for the UK government's ozone conference in London in March 1989—to try to encourage the uncommitted countries to sign up. Frankly, if countries like China and India do not sign the Protocol and do achieve the basic level of one refrigerator per household, their use will be as much as in the rest of the world now, and our efforts to reduce the use of CFCs in aerosols and polyurethane foams, etc. will have been negated.

There is already much discussion about whether the Protocol measures are sufficient. It is under review this year, with decisions to be made in the spring of 1990. The freeze will stay because the freeze will already have happened. I do not think the timing can be advanced significantly, but the percentage reductions might be greater. I can foresee the 50% cut moved forward a few years and replaced by an 85 to 90% cut by the end of the century. In fact the UK government is committed to a minimum 85% cutback by the end of the century.

Does it make any difference how soon the Protocol is made more stringent? Basically, no, apart from public relations value, as is shown in Fig. 5. The vertical scale is parts per billion (ppb) of chlorine in the atmosphere. This is purely chlorine from CFCs; natural chlorine has been ignored. The top line, A, is what happens if the Protocol is followed— that is, how chlorine from CFCs will continue to increase in the atmosphere from the current level of less than 2 ppb to 4 ppb—it will virtually double. If the Protocol is advanced marginally, i.e., we have a 20% cut this year and a 50% cut in 1993, it does not make a lot of difference, (Line B). The reason is the long lifetime of CFCs in the atmosphere. It takes a long time for them to reach steady-state concentration. Most dramatic would be a 95% cut this year, which would cause chlorine in the atmosphere to follow Line F. But a 95% cut now is not on: there are too many important uses for that to be feasible. Supposing we take the freeze as planned, the 20 and 50% cuts as planned, and then a 95% cut just after the turn of the century, shown by Line D. It is clear we are now talking about differences of fractions of a part per billion of chlorine in the atmosphere. An 85% cut this year is not feasible, but the span of the four options is about half a ppb. Compared with the Protocol as written, it really does not make a lot of difference, but there is an enormous difference in impact on the user industries.

Figure 6 shows the approximate world usage of CFCs in 1986, the Montreal Protocol base year. The actual pattern of use varies very widely between different areas of the world. In the USA, for instance, where use of aerosols has been largely eliminated, refrigeration and air conditioning is a very major use. In Europe, the aerosol industry still represents about 50% of the market, but is declining fast. The European aerosol industry has adopted a target of reducing its use of CFCs by around 90% by the end of this year. It is that sort of figure that enables the Government to say we will have achieved a 50% cutback next year. The aerosol industry will have done it for them. In fact, the pressure is on every other industry to minimize their use, and in particular to minimize its *losses* of CFCs.

In terms of per capita use, the EEC and United States are near one kilo per annum. If India and China were conceivably to rise to this level, their usage would swamp the rest of the world. Of course, use in India and China is never going to approach that because I

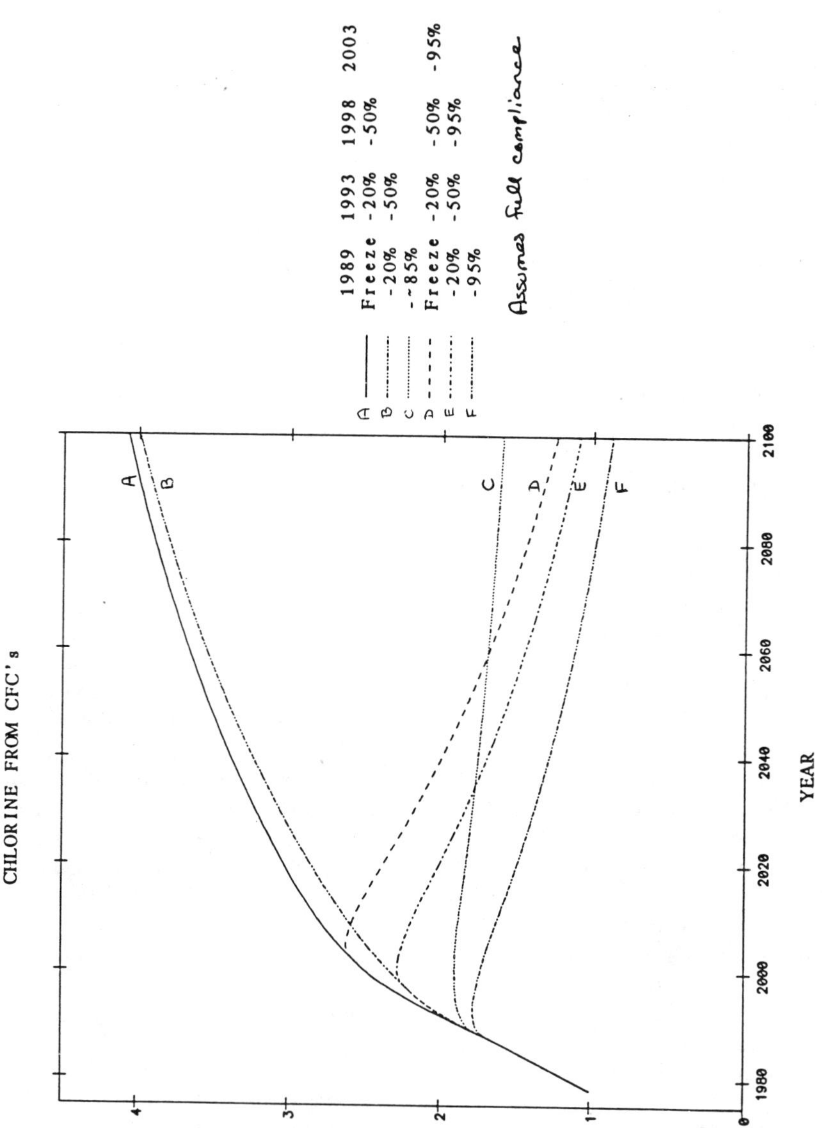

FIG. 5—*Future estimates of the effects from chlorine from CFCs with different international regulatory strategies.*

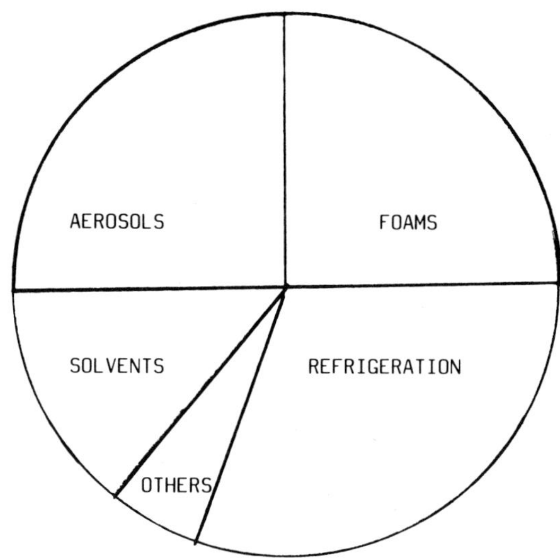

FIG. 6—*Estimated 1986 CFCs usage. Approximate world total is 1 100 000 tons.*

cannot see those countries developing aerosol industries that use CFCs in the way the western world has.

For Russia we have numbers up to the mid-70s, but then they stopped providing the data. For a while we extrapolated at the same growth rate, but the numbers began to get unwieldy. Russian production is probably around 100 000 tons—but that is a guess.

We are now looking for alternatives to the CFCs. Figure 7 gives an idea of the range of compounds that have been looked at as potential alternatives to the regulated CFCs. Some have chlorine, some have no chlorine, but they all contain hydrogen and fluorine so we call them hydrofluoroalkanes (HFAs). Will these alternatives be better? The most likely ones, shown in Fig. 8, are HFAs 123, 134a, and 141b. HFA 134a has no chlorine and hence cannot have any impact on ozone. HFAs 123 and 141b have chlorine and could in theory survive into the stratosphere. But the key to it is that they contain hydrogen. One attempt has been made at computer calculating their ozone depletion potential (ODP), and Figure 9 shows predictions of different computer models. CFCs 11 and 12 for all practical purposes have an ozone depletion of 1, an arbitrary number. ODPs for the other three regulated materials, 113, 114, and 115, range downwards from 0.8 to 0.6.

Then we come to the hydrogen-containing materials, labelled HFA. Those not containing chlorine clearly have no ODP, but those that have chlorine show a contribution to ozone depletion of only one tenth to one twentieth that of fully halogenated materials. The reason comes down to bond energies. Figure 10 shows the strengths of the various bonds: carbon-carbon, carbon-oxygen, carbon-hydrogen, bromine, chlorine, and fluorine. Look at the strength of the carbon-fluorine bond compared with that for carbon-chlorine and carbon-hydrogen. In a molecule that is only carbon, chlorine, and fluorine, it is chlorine that is going to split off. In a molecule that has carbon, chlorine, and hydrogen, both chlorine and hydrogen provide a form of weakness, with the hydrogen leading to reaction with hydroxyl (OH′) radicals in the troposphere.

I included oxygen because some anesthetics contain oxygen. Figure 11 shows the resemblance, particular with halothane, with one or two of the alternatives to CFCs that we are looking at. This underlines one of the problems we have already encountered in doing animal toxicity testing with one of the alternatives: it is a very good anesthetic. At the

	CFCs		FCs
21	$CHCl_2F$	23	CHF_3
22	$CHClF_2$	32	CH_2F_2
31	CH_2ClF	41	CH_3F
121	$CHCl_2\text{-}CCl_2F$	125	$CHF_2\text{-}CF_3$
122a	$CHClF\text{-}CCl_2F$	134a	$CH_2F\text{-}CF_3$
123	$CHCl_2\text{-}CF_3$	143	$CH_2F\text{-}CHF_2$
124a	$CHF_2\text{-}CClF_2$	152a	$CH_3\text{-}CHF_2$
131	$CHCl_2\text{-}CHClF$	161	$CH_3\text{-}CH_2F$
132b	$CH_2Cl\text{-}CClF_2$	227	$CHF_2\text{-}CF_2\text{-}CF_3$
133a	$CH_2Cl\text{-}CF_3$	236	$CHF_2\text{-}CF_2\text{-}CHF_2$
142b	$CH_3\text{-}CClF_2$	272	$CH_2F\text{-}CH_2\text{-}CH_2F$
151	$CH_2Cl\text{-}CH_2F$	C 216	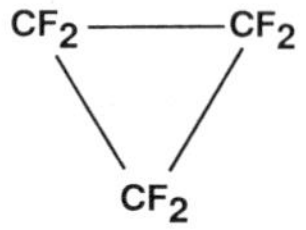 CF_2————CF_2
226	$CHF_2\text{-}CCl_2\text{-}CF_3$		(cyclic, with CF_2)
262	$CH_2Cl\text{-}CH_2\text{-}CHF_2$		CF_2

FIG. 7—*More than 40 compounds were in the first listing of possible substitutes.*

Potential CFC Alternatives

CF_3CHCl_2	dichlorotrifluoromethane	HFA 123
$CFCl_2CH_3$	dichlorofluoroethane	HFA 141b
CF_3CH_2F	tetrafluoroethane	HFA 134a

FIG. 8—*Potential CFC alternatives.*

highest dose levels, 5% in air, the animals fell asleep. Enflurane and isoflurane are significantly different in that they have a carbon-oxygen linkup. The presence of C-O and C-H bonds explains why the halogenated anesthetics cannot have the same impact on ozone as the fully saturated CFCs. Chemically, they are sufficiently similar to the hydrofluoroalkane alternatives, which have only 5 to 10% of the potential for depleting ozone compared with the fully halogenated CFCs.

The other factor is tonnage production, and CFCs 11 and 12 are by far the major compounds. Taking all the CFCs together, we are close on a million tons per annum at the moment. If you take the halogenated anesthetics together, the total is about one thousand tons, giving a factor of a thousand times between the halogenated anesthetics and the CFCs. Add that to the much-reduced potential for ozone depletion, by analogy with the alternatives the industry is looking at, and you can put the possible role of halogenated anesthetics in global ozone depletion into perspective.

To give some sort of numerical perspective to this talk of a thousand or a million tons per annum, roughly 30 million tons of ozone are produced and destroyed by natural stratospheric processes every day.

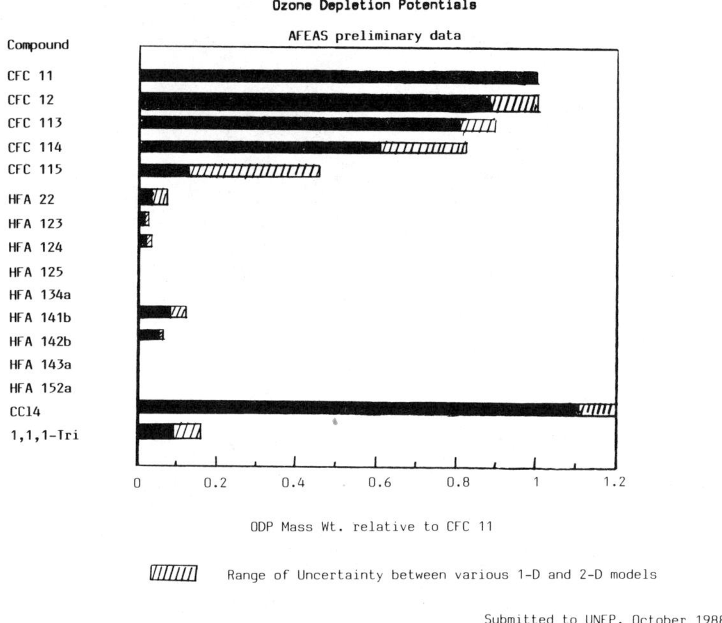

FIG. 9—*Ozone depletion potentials—AFEAS preliminary data.*

Bond Energies

	kg. cal. / mole
C-C	58.6
C-O	70.0
C-H	87.3
C-Br	54.0
C-Cl	66.5
C-F	107.0
H-Cl	102.7
H-F	147.5

FIG. 10—*Bond energies.*

Going on to the greenhouse effect, energy comes from the sun as ultraviolet radiation, is absorbed by the earth, and reemitted in the infrared waveband. Various gases in the atmosphere absorb a proportion of the energy emitted from the earth's surface and, in effect, reflect it back. This creates a habitable climate. If we did not have a greenhouse effect, we would not have life as we know it. It is what makes the difference between a temperature which would be 20 to 30° subzero and the temperature of roughly 20°C that we enjoy. This absorption is principally due to water vapor and carbon dioxide in the atmosphere with contributions from methane, nitrous oxide, and CFCs.

Why do these gases absorb? Essentially, infrared radiation emitted from the earth escapes through an atmospheric window, at 7 to 13 μm, where there is a particularly low absorption by water vapor. Water vapor absorbs all the way along the spectrum, but with varying intensity, and in this window there is little. The window is partly filled by carbon dioxide,

HFAs and Halogenated Anaesthetics

HFA 123	$CF_3 - CHCl_2$
HFA 134a	$CF_3 - CH_2F$
HFA 141b	$CFCl_2 - CH_3$
Halothane	$CF_3 - CHClBr$
Enflurane	$CHClF - CF_2 - O - CHF_2$
Isoflurane	$CF_3 - CHCl - O - CHF_2$

FIG. 11—*HFAs and halogenated anesthetics.*

which overlaps, but other gases also absorb within this window. These gases are principally man-made, but include also methane and nitrous oxide.

Every bit of absorption in that window theoretically adds to the greenhouse effect, reducing the emission of heat that would normally escape, *in theory* raising the temperature of the earth. I say in theory because scientists themselves are undecided as to the extent of any warming (there is even a minor school of thought that says there will be a greenhouse cooling), and, if there is one, what the effect will be. As the atmosphere warms up, will we get greater evaporation of water from the oceans and hence more cloud cover, which will absorb radiation—preventing it coming in and preventing it going out? The whole question is extremely complicated.

Over the last hundred years, it is estimated there has been a warming of about 0.5°C, the bulk of which has happened in the last 20 to 30 years. Whether that will continue is anyone's guess. But, assuming it does, how will the various greenhouse gases contribute? Figure 12 shows the relative contributions of the various gases projected to 2030. The CO_2 and methane contributions will double over that period at present rates of emission, nitrous oxide will increase by around three times, CFCs will have doubled but will already be beginning to decline as the Montreal Protocol measures take effect.

With at least half of the warming coming from carbon dioxide, this is the area where the most attention should be devoted. A large part of it comes from the burning of fossil fuels. The crux must be improved energy efficiency. If we are going to continue burning fossil fuels to produce energy, the answer must be to make maximum use of every ton of carbon burned.

Nitrous oxide arises from various agricultural (but not necessarily man-induced) activities. Methane likewise comes from agricultural practices, from rotting vegetation, as in rice paddies and tropical forests, and from all grass-eating animals who generate large amounts of methane in their digestive systems, and hence can be affected by changes in farming practice. The combined contribution from CFCs and their replacements, HFAs, is less than 15% of the total.

The figures on nitrous oxide are based on a World Meteorological Organization report in 1985 [4]. The current atmospheric loading of nitrous oxide was 2350 million tons. The contributions to that—these are very approximate—are 2 million tons annually from the oceans, 5 million tons from burning coal and oil, and 1 million tons from other biomass burning such as slash and burn agriculture.

Agricultural practices themselves, nitrogenous fertilizers breaking down in the soil, contributed a little less than 1 million tons, natural processes on grassland about a tenth of that, forest and woodland in temperate zones about 500 000 tons, and tropical forests 8 million tons.

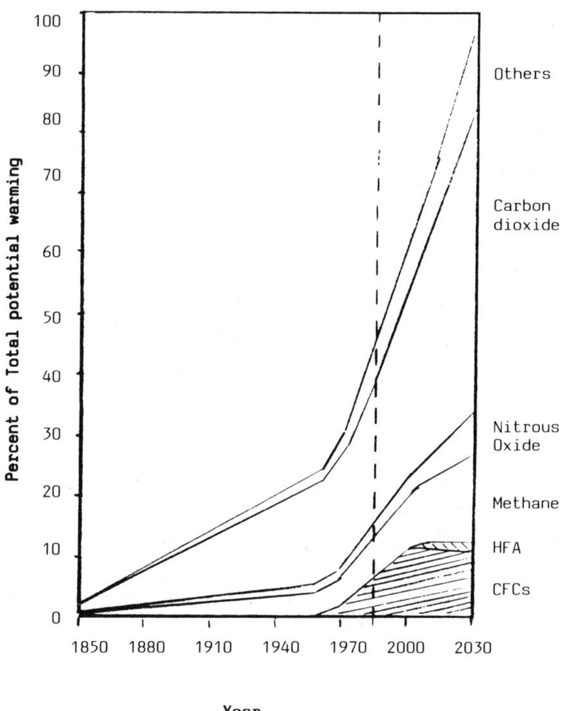

FIG. 12—*Relative contributions to greenhouse effect (based on WMO report of 1985).*

About 14 million tons are used up in various ways in the atmosphere, leaving a growth of about 3 million tons per annum on a total burden of 2300 million tons. Set against that we have anesthetic use. I am indebted to Dr. Bray for the UK nitrous oxide usage, which I converted to tons. I assumed that the UK represents 10% of the world's anesthesia practice, so I have taken a world figure of 20 000 tons—compared with the millions of tons we are talking about.

I do not mean that we should forget the problem and gleefully vent everything to the atmosphere, but when you are dealing with nitrogen oxides in an airstream you have to catalytically convert them. It is not as simple as scrubbing, but it is not impossible. But really it is a counsel of perfection. As a contribution, it is very small. If the anesthetics industry wants to be seen doing something, then the possibility of catalytic converters on the exhaust systems of major hospitals might be worth considering. But it is not going to make a significant difference.

References

[1] Rowland, F. S. and Molina, M. J., "Chlorofluoromethanes in the Environment," AEC Report 1974-1, University of California, Irvine, CA, September 1974.
[2] Dobson, G. M. B. and Harrison, D. N., *Proceedings of the Royal Society of London, Series A, Mathematical and Physical Sciences*, Vol. 110, 1 Apr. 1926, pp. 660–693.
[3] Schneider, S. H., *Science*, Vol. 243, 10 Feb. 1989, pp. 771–781.
[4] World Meteorological Organization, "Atmospheric Ozone 1985, Assessment of Our Understanding of the Process Controlling Its Present Distribution and Change," NASA, Washington, DC, 1986.
[5] Scotto, J., Cotton, G., Urbach, F., Berger, D., and Fears, T., *Science*, Vol. 239, 12 Feb. 1988, pp. 762–764.

Jan-Peter A. H. Jantzen[1]

Anestheticography: Clinical Applications

REFERENCE: Jantzen, J.- P. A. H., **"Anestheticography: Clinical Applications,"** *Continuous Anesthesia Gas Monitoring, ASTM STP 1090,* J. Hedley-Whyte and P. W. Thompson, Eds., American Society for Testing and Materials, Philadelphia, 1990, pp. 47–52.

ABSTRACT: The safe practice of inhalation anesthesia requires control over the amount of volatile anesthetic delivered to the patient. This is facilitated by continuous monitoring and recording of the agents' concentration ("anestheticography"). Either the vaporizer or the circuit may be considered the "delivery system," hence anestheticometry performed either in the fresh gas supply or in the inspiratory limb of the system is acceptable. Such monitoring practice may be expected to eliminate anesthesia-related death due to overdose of volatile agents. Besides the aspects of technical safety, anestheticometry is a useful adjunct to teaching and research. It supports a more widespread application of the minimal-flow and closed-circuit techniques, facilitates the understanding of inhalation anesthesia, and increases acceptance of low-flow systems. For minimal-flow anesthesia, anestheticometry should be considered mandatory because it provides the only means of detecting and correcting derangements of the anesthetic vapor concentration, often brought about by routine clinical maneuvers.

To demonstrate this, we recorded the course of the inspiratory and expiratory concentration of a volatile anesthetic (isoflurane) by infrared absorption and a trend recorder. Changing the carrier gas composition during high flow (fresh gas flow = 6.0 L·min^{-1}) from 75 to 25 vol % nitrous oxide in oxygen resulted in a 10% increase of the inspiratory isoflurane concentration. Activating the oxygen bypass or exchanging the soda lime canisters was followed by a prolonged reduction of concentration, most pronounced with minimal flow (fresh gas flow = 0.5 L·min^{-1}). Initiating emergence by closing the vaporizer during minimal flow led to a slow decrease in concentration, while at high flow the inspiratory isoflurane concentration rapidly decreased to subanesthetic levels. Integration of a charcoal filter into the inspiratory limb of the breathing circuit reduces the inspiratory concentration to undetectable levels within <3 min. Anestheticography is a useful means of monitoring and documentation of inhalation anesthetic. Such monitoring should become part of ISO standards for reasons of patient safety, economy, teaching, and research.

KEY WORDS: monitoring, anesthetic vapors, concentration, anesthesia, inhalation, minimal flow technique, equipment, infrared analyzer, charcoal filter

If one compares the inhalation route of administration with the intravenous route, with the latter there is the advantage of knowing exactly what has been administered to the patient. This is not the case with a volatile agent because the patient will expire a certain proportion of what he has received. A major advantage, however, of the inhalation agent is that one can continuously determine what is inside the patient at a given moment by means of end-tidal anestheticometry. Ten or 20 samples may be analyzed each minute, which certainly would be difficult with any intravenous drug regimen.

The inherent safety element of measuring the amount of potent drugs delivered to a patient prompted the German federal government to make the continuous monitoring of volatile anesthetic agents compulsatory. Effective 1 January 1988, the Medical Apparatus Safety Act (Medizingeräteverordnung) requires all new anesthesia machines be equipped

[1]Associate professor of anesthesiology, Department of Anaesthesiology, Johannes Gutenberg-University Medical School, Mainz, Federal Republic of Germany.

with an anestheticometer, which monitors the volatile agents' concentration either at the common gas outlet or in the inspiratory limb, including the Y-piece. Subsequent to a recent case of massive halothane overdose evolving from a vaporizer malfunction and resulting in permanent brain damage to a child and a law suit, a number of state authorities and hospital administrations in Germany have extended this monitor requirement to include all older equipment, too.

The safe practice of inhalation anesthesia depends on accurate control of the amount of volatile anesthetic delivered to the patient. Errors may lead to serious consequences [1,2]. With high flows into circle systems or nonrebreathing systems, the vaporizer's dial setting provides sufficient information. However, with minimal flows into closed circuit systems, the inspiratory concentration of the volatile agent is less predictable [3] and should be monitored [4]. While continuous monitoring of the CO_2 concentration (capnometry) and its graphic presentation (capnography) are well established techniques [5,6], the measurement of anesthetic gases and vapors was introduced into clinical practice only recently. In clinical settings this is performed mainly by four techniques: mass spectrometry [7], piezoelectric resonance [8], infrared absorption [9–11], and Raman spectroscopy [12].

Mass spectrometry is the most accurate. However, the systems available are too expensive for broad clinical application. Based on the infrared absorption principle, the IRINA™ (Dräger) measures halothane, enflurane, isoflurane, and nitrous oxide in either the inspiratory or expiratory limb of a circuit (mainstream). This device is the only commercially available infrared absorption spectrometer capable of identifying volatile anesthetics and their mixtures. The Normac™ and the Capnomac™ (Datex) measure halothane, enflurane, and isoflurane by continuous sampling from the Y-piece or the inspiratory or expiratory limb of the circuit (sidestream). The sample gas can be returned to the circuit. Satisfactory performance of the Normac was recently proven [9–11].

Minimal flow technique is defined as a rebreathing system with a fresh gas flow of <500 mL·min^{-1} [13]. With respect to airway humidification and cost effectiveness, the advantages of this technique are documented [14–17]. Nevertheless, its use is not widespread, chiefly because of the unpredictability of the actual inspiratory concentration of the anesthetic agent at the lower flow rates [3].

Another drawback is the prolonged emergence due to a slow washout of the anesthetic. This can be overcome by the use of an activated charcoal filter, a simple but effective method described earlier [18].

We evaluated whether graphical presentation of the anesthetic's concentration aids in interpretation of changes caused by various clinical situations during minimal- and high-flow anesthesia and how an activated charcoal filter affects anesthetic concentration, N_2O, and circuit climate.

Materials and Methods

We used a Normac infrared absorption monitor to follow the course of anesthetic gas concentrations in a rebreathing system based on an AV-1™ anesthesia machine (Dräger) equipped with an isoflurane vaporizer (Vapor 19-1™, Dräger). Both devices proved suitable for minimal flow technique [19,20]. Documentation was with a modified two-channel trend recorder (Dräger). The scale was adjusted to 1 vol % = 40 mm and the speed set at 10 mm·min^{-1}. Isoflurane (I) was the anesthetic used (inspiratory concentration: F_iI, expiratory concentration: $F_{ex}I$). Minimal-, high-, and wash-out flow was defined as a fresh gas flow of 0.5, 3.0, and 6.0 L·min^{-1}, respectively.

A coal filter was assembled from an autoclavable plastic container with ISO adapters (Servo-Humidifier 150™, Siemens), activated charcoal (Charcoal Activated Granular 2.5 mm™, Merck), and a surgical gauze swab. This filter was mounted either upstream or downstream from the CO_2 absorbent canister.

The following situations frequently encountered in clinical routine were recorded:

1. Changing the carrier gas composition from 25 to 75 vol % O_2 in N_2O and then to 35 vol % O_2 in N_2 at high flow.
2. Activating the oxygen bypass for 10 s (35 L·min^{-1}) during high and minimal flow.
3. Exchanging both soda lime canisters during high and minimal flow.
4. Terminating administration of the volatile anesthetic by closing the vaporizer, and

    a. Maintaining minimal flow.
    b. Changing to washout flow.
    c. Inserting a charcoal filter during minimal flow either upstream from the soda lime canister, or:
    d. Downstream from the soda lime canister.

Figures 1 to 3 represent original recordings.

Results

1. A change of the carrier gas composition from 25 to 75 vol % O_2 in N_2O, while maintaining a high flow with the vaporizer dial set at 1.5 vol % resulted in a 10% increase of the recorded F_iI. A subsequent change to oxygen in room air (O_2 35 vol %) resulted in a slight decrease of the inspired isoflurane concentration.
2. Flushing the system with the oxygen bypass (35 L·min^{-1}) for 10 s resulted in a sudden drop and a long-lasting derangement of concentration. During high flow, F_iI fell by 35% and took >10 min to recover. With minimal flow this led to a drop of F_iI by 50% and a recovery time of >25 min (Fig. 1).
3. Similar effects were created by changing the soda lime canisters. During high flow F_iI dropped by more than 80%, with minimal flow F_iI transiently dropped to zero in some patients. Recovery took >8 and >20 min, respectively (Fig. 2).
4. Washout of the volatile anesthetic is flow dependent.

    a. Closing the vaporizer and maintaining minimal flow resulted in a delayed decrease in concentration. A fall of the inspiratory isoflurane concentration from 0.7 to 0.15 vol % took >1 h.

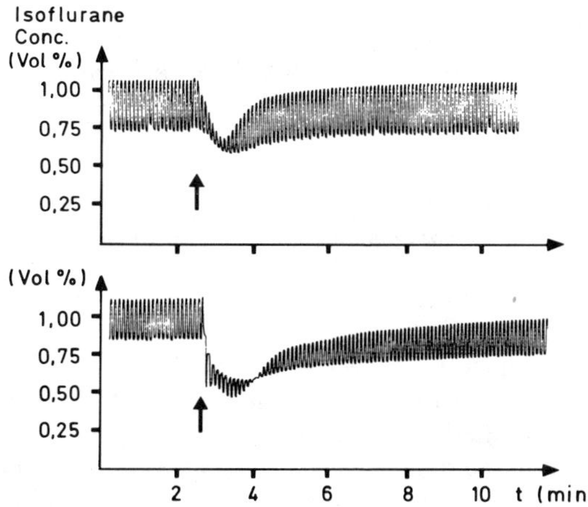

FIG. 1—*Effects of activating the oxygen bypass for 10 s (marker) during high flow (above) and minimal flow (below).*

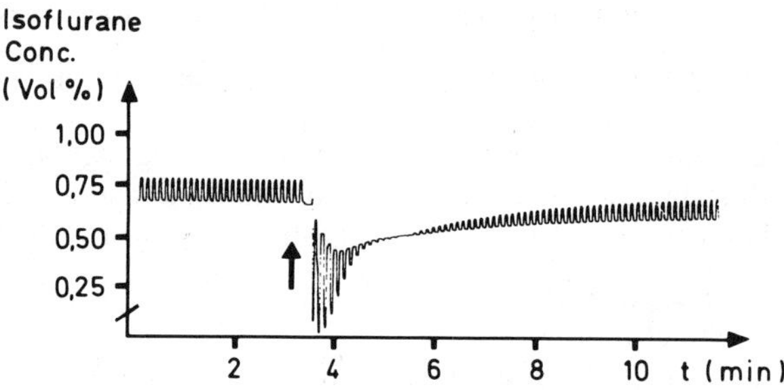

FIG. 2—*Effects of exchanging both soda lime canisters (marker) during minimal flow.*

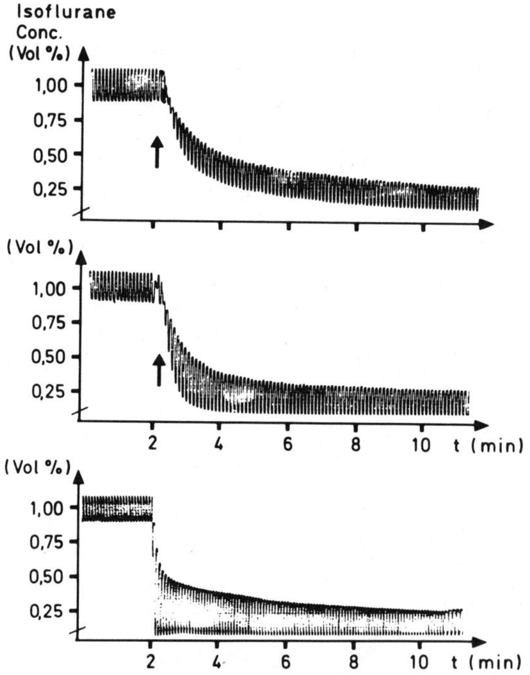

FIG. 3—*Effects of closing the vaporizer (marker):* upper curve: *increasing the fresh gas flow rate to 6 L·min⁻¹;* middle: *maintaining minimal flow and integrating an activated charcoal filter upstream from the soda lime canister;* bottom: *idem, but mounting the filter downstream from the soda lime.*

b. With washout flow this was achieved within 5 min.

c., d. The integration of an activated charcoal filter into the circuit reduced F_iI to zero within 3 min when mounted upstream, and within one ventilatory cycle when mounted downstream from the soda lime canister (Fig. 3). This filter did not absorb moisture or adsorb nitrous oxide to alter these parameters, nor did it influence inspiratory gas temperature.

Discussion

The end-tidal concentration of a volatile anesthetic (Et_{VA}) was recently shown to be the closest alternative to brain concentration [21], making on-line monitoring of Et_{VA} a desirable asset to inhalation anesthesia.

We used "anestheticography" in a clinical setting based on an AV 1 anesthesia machine (Dräger) and an infrared absorption anestheticometer (Normac, Datex).

F_iI was altered by more than 10% by changing the carrier gas composition alone. The highest F_iI was achieved with oxygen, closely followed by nitrogen, and by far the lowest values were seen with nitrous oxide. Thus, turning off the nitrous oxide while keeping the total fresh gas flow and the vaporizer setting constant will increase the amount of volatile anesthetic delivered to the patient. This may have a potentially lethal effect [22]. The increase is partly due to the lower viscosity and kinematic viscosity of N_2O, resulting in the lowest critical velocity [23] and partly to a different solubility of the carrier gas in the volatile anesthetic [22,24]. However, interpretation of this observation must consider an inaccuracy of the Normac readings in the range of 6 to 8% when higher concentrations of N_2O are used [9,11].

Activating the oxygen bypass delivers a huge amount (35 L·min^{-1}) of anesthetic-free gas into the circuit. This results in a sharp reduction of F_iI and subsequently of $F_{ex}I$. Following 10 s of O_2 flushing, recovery to control ranged from 10 to 30 min, depending on the fresh gas flow rate (Fig. 1). Graphical presentation of this effect aids in rapidly restoring the desired anesthetic concentration by modifying the vaporizer dial setting or fresh gas flow. The same holds true for another "disturbance" experienced in clinical routine. Exchange of the soda lime canisters affects the vapor concentration by two mechanisms. Besides soda lime, one set of canisters contains approximately 1.5 L of room air, thus diluting the gas mixture in the circuit. This causes a sudden decrease. Secondly, dry soda lime will adsorb a significant amount of isoflurane [25]. This is a possible explanation for the longer recovery times following soda lime exchange, compared to those following oxygen flushing. These changes are more pronounced with minimal flow.

For termination of anesthesia, a rapid decrease of the inspired vapor concentration is desirable. In a rebreathing system, the turnover rate is dependent upon fresh gas flow rate. Thus, shutting off the vaporizer and maintaining a minimal flow results in unacceptably long washout times. Currently, the only option is to increase fresh gas flow, thus changing to a nonrebreathing system. A washout flow of 6 L·min^{-1} will reduce F_iI to inspiratory concentrations of <0.2 vol % within 5 min.

Integration of a charcoal filter into the circuit affects F_iI rapidly, reducing it to zero within 3 min, independent of fresh gas flow. Elimination will be the faster, the smaller the apparatus dead space (buffer volume) between the charcoal and the tracheal tube becomes. Thus, integration of the filter downstream from the soda lime canister resulted in an elimination of isoflurane from the inspiratory gas mixture within one ventilatory cycle (Fig. 3). This device provides a means for rapid emergence while maintaining the merits of minimal flow. The principle of adsorption of anesthetic vapors onto activated charcoal was pioneered by Tiegel and Dräger in 1934 [26], rediscovered by Epstein and Berlin in 1944 [27], and subsequently has found wide application in scavenging systems. However, its use to reduce anesthetic concentration in circuit systems was suggested only a decade ago [18]. Such a filter may be made from materials available in most hospitals, rendering it both cheap and reusable [26,28–30]. Recently, its use was recommended to "decontaminate" an anesthesia circuit from vapors in case of malignant hyperthermia [31]. Our evaluation of this filter in a clinical setting proved its effectiveness in rapidly eliminating isoflurane from the inspiratory gas mixture. The filter was found to alter neither temperature nor humidity or to adsorb nitrous oxide.

Conclusions

After three years of routine clinical application we conclude that "anestheticography" is an informative and noninvasive asset to monitoring and documentation and contributes to a better understanding of inhalation anesthesia. It facilitates interpretation and correction of derangements in gas composition, thus rendering the minimal flow technique both easier and safer.

The activated charcoal filter reliably adsorbs volatile agents, thus allowing minimal flow throughout the entire anesthetic, including emergence.

References

[1] Doblar, D. D. and Hinkle, I. C., *Anesthesiology*, Vol. 61, 1984, pp. 220–222.
[2] Martin, S. T., *Anesthesiology*, Vol. 62, 1985, pp. 830–831.
[3] Baer, B., *Anaesthesist*, Vol. 32, 1983, pp. 6–11.
[4] Schwilden, H., *Anästhesie, Intensivtherapie, Notfallmedizin*, Vol. 20, 1985, pp. 307–315.
[5] Lenz, G., Klöss, T., and Schorer, R., *Anästhesiologie und Intensivmedizin*, Vol. 26, 1985, pp. 133–141.
[6] Smalhout, B. and Kalenda, Z., *An Atlas of Capnography*, Zeist, Kerckebosch, The Netherlands, 1975.
[7] Lichtiger, M., *Seminars in Anesthesia*, Vol. 5, 1985, pp. 206–212.
[8] Hayes, J. K., Westenskow, D. R., and Jordan, W. S., *Anesthesiology*, Vol. 59, 1983, pp. 435–439.
[9] Colquhoun, A. D., Gray, W. M., and Asbury, A. J., *Anaesthesia*, Vol. 41, 1986, pp. 198–204.
[10] Luff, N. P. and White, D. C., *Anaesthesia*, Vol. 40, 1985, p. 555–559.
[11] Zbinden, A. M., Westenskow, D. R., Thomson, D. A., Funk, B., and Maertens, J., *International Journal of Clinical Monitoring and Computing*, Vol. 2, 1986, pp. 151–161.
[12] Westenskow, D. R., Smith, K. W., Coleman, D. C., Gregonis, D. E., and Van Wagenen, R. A., *Anesthesiology*, Vol. 70, 1989, pp. 350–355.
[13] Baum, J. and Schneider, U., *Anästhesiologie und Intensivmedizin*, Vol. 24, 1983, pp. 263–269.
[14] Aldrete, J. A., Cubillos, P., and Sherrill, D., *Acta Anaesthesiologica Scandinavica*, Vol. 25, 1981, pp. 312–314.
[15] Droh, R., and Rothmann, G., *Anaesthesist*, Vol. 26, 1977, pp. 461–466.
[16] Droh, R., Rolly, G., and Schepp, R., *Acta Anaesthesiologica Belgica*, Vol. 35, 1984, pp. 265–272.
[17] Rayburn, R. L., and Watson, R. L., *Anesthesiology*, Vol. 52, 1980, pp. 291–295.
[18] Bushman, J. A., Enderby, D. H., Al-Abrak, M. H., and Askill, S., *British Journal of Anaesthesia*, Vol. 49, 1977, pp. 575–587.
[19] Lin, C. Y., *Anesthesia and Analgesia*, Vol. 59, 1980, pp. 359–366.
[20] Rolly, G. and Versichelen, L., *Acta Anaesthesiologica Belgica*, Vol. 35, 1984, pp. 329–341.
[21] Zbinden, A. M., Frei, F., Westenskow, D. R., and Thomson, D. A., *British Journal of Anaesthesia*, Vol. 58, 1986, pp. 563–571.
[22] Scheller, M. S. and Drummond, J. C., *Anesthesia and Analgesia*, Vol. 65, 1986, pp. 88–90.
[23] Palayiwa, E., Sanderson, M. H., and Hahn, C. E. W., *British Journal of Anaesthesia*, Vol. 55, 1983, pp. 1025–1038.
[24] Gould, D. B., Lampert, B. A., and MacKrell, T. N., *Anesthesia and Analgesia*, Vol. 61, 1982, pp. 938–940.
[25] Grodin, W. K., Epstein, M. A. F. and Epstein, R. A., *Anesthesiology*, Vol. 62, 1985, pp. 60–64.
[26] Jantzen, J.-P. A. H. and Kleemann, P. P., *Fortschritte der Anaesthesiologie*, Vol. 2, 1988, pp. 56–63.
[27] Epstein, H. G. and Berlin, D. P., *Lancet*, Vol. 1, 1944, pp. 114–116.
[28] Baumgarten, R. K., *Anesthesiology*, Vol. 63, 1985, p. 125.
[29] Ernst, E. A., *Anesthesiology*, Vol. 57, 1982, p. 343.
[30] Jantzen, J.-P. A. H., *Anesthesiology*, Vol. 69, 1988, pp. 437–438.
[31] Greene, E. R., *Anesthesiology*, Vol. 65, 1986, p. 420.

Clive S. Bray[1]

Economics of Anesthetic Gas Monitoring

REFERENCE: Bray, C. S., **"Economics of Anesthetic Gas Monitoring,"** *Continuous Anesthesia Gas Monitoring, ASTM STP 1090*, J. Hedley-Whyte and P. W. Thompson, Eds., American Society for Testing and Materials, Philadelphia, 1990, pp. 53–59.

ABSTRACT: The purpose of this paper is to attempt to identify and quantify the cost differences in the United Kingdom (UK) between continuous-flow open anesthetic systems and low-flow closed systems. Due to the lack of reliable statistics, such an appraisal is difficult, and at best this paper can give only a likely indication of the actual costs involved. Costs will vary significantly from country to country, and a detailed study for any particular site is necessary if meaningful results are to be obtained.

Annual running costs for Raman laser, infrared, and piezoelectric type monitors have been estimated. A significant expense is the provision of the disposable gas sampling line, if it is changed in accordance with the manufacturer's recommended intervals.

An estimate is made of the money spent on volatile agents and anesthetic gases in the UK, and the potential savings from decreasing gas flow from 10 to 2 L/min. is also estimated. These figures are compared with the estimated cost of providing all operating theatres in the UK with anesthetic gas monitoring equipment.

Other factors such as additional expenditure on soda lime and savings on other monitoring equipment, e.g., oxygen analyzers, are taken into account.

The Pharmaceutical Price Regulation Scheme is briefly explained, as well as the likely effect of the scheme on savings in the use of volatile agents.

KEY WORDS: anesthesia, gases, monitoring, economics, equipment, consumables

The purpose of this paper is to attempt to identify and quantify the costs associated with continuous-flow open system anesthesia and to compare these costs with those of low-flow systems.

Because of the lack of reliable statistics, certain assumptions are made, and the figures provided should be used only as a likely indication of the actual costs involved. In order to determine the economic benefits of any particular system, a full on-site analysis needs to be performed. Figure 1 shows the cost of commonly used volatile agents in various countries.

All costs quoted in this paper are in pounds sterling, and as far as can be ascertained are those incurred by a typical UK hospital. That is not necessarily the manufacturer's quoted price: costs to the National Health Service (NHS) are often significantly cheaper.

It was not possible to calculate the costs of anesthetics gases and volatile agents for an individual hospital without a detailed and time-consuming study. However, a total UK figure for these commodities is known, and the economic calculations are based on these data.

Assumptions

Because of a lack of reliable statistics, it is necessary to make a number of assumptions:

1. An identical anesthetic machine can be used for either open- or closed-system anesthesia, and therefore the costs are the same for either case. Furthermore, although the

[1]Superintendent, Product Group 1, Supplies Technology Division, Department of Health, London, United Kingdom.

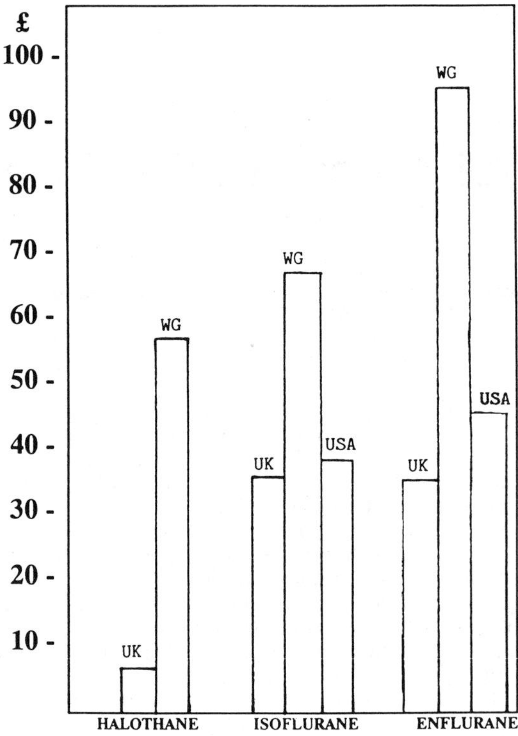

FIG. 1—*Comparison of cost of volatile agents (per bottle) in the United Kingdom, West Germany, and the United States.*

breathing system will have a different configuration, the cost of provision of either type will not be significantly different.

2. The anesthetic machine used for open-system anesthesia is provided with an oxygen analyzer.

3. Costs are based on amortizing the initial equipment cost over a five-year period. In this period it is assumed that the equipment will be serviced by the manufacturer and that no additional costs are incurred (i.e., there are no component replacements other than those covered in the servicing arrangements). It is assumed that any disposable item, e.g., sampling gas line, is used in accordance with the manufacturer's instructions and is provided by the manufacturer. The cost of such items is based, initially, on one disposable per session, i.e., 500 per annum. For some types of monitor, the consumption of electricity adds significantly to the running cost. Electricity is charged to the NHS at £0.039 per kWh, and electricity costs are calculated on 2500 h per annum.

It is a fairly simple job to calculate the running cost of a particular item of equipment for a twelve-month period, but in order to make a comparison with the annual figures for usage of anesthetic agents it is necessary to convert the running cost into an annual national figure. Thus it is necessary to multiply the individual cost by the number of units in use. The figure of 3500 has been used for this purpose.

Because of the lack of readily available data, a further assumption has been made with regard to the theoretical versus the actual savings that will be achieved in reduction of gas usage. Typically an open system utilizes a total gas flow for an adult of between 8 to 10 L per minute, whereas a closed system will use somewhere between $\frac{1}{2}$ and 3 L/min. Clearly a reduction in flow from say 10 to 2 L/min creates a theoretical saving of 80%. However, in practice it is found that savings are significantly less. The reasons for this are as follows:

1. The patient will require the same quantity of gas and anesthetic agent during induction and the early stages of anesthesia.
2. The patient will require the same quantity of oxygen during the recovery period.

Thus savings can only be achieved during the steady state, and long procedures provide the greatest potential for cost savings. Assessment of the actual saving was difficult in the available time, but I was able to find one paper that dealt with actual rather than theoretical savings. This was published in *Anaesthesiology* in 1987 and gives data from the University of Maryland. The paper indicates that a reduction in fresh gas flow from between 3 to 5 to 1 to 2 L/min resulted in an actual saving of about 40% (theoretical saving is about 60%). Other papers I found generally indicated that significant cost reductions were possible and gave some indication of the theoretical savings, but were unable to confirm these. In the absence of other suitable data, I have therefore used the 40% figure as an achievable value for the purpose of this paper.

Areas of Cost Saving

If these assumptions are accepted, then cost savings due to the following can be considered:

1. Reduction in use of volatile agents.
2. Reduction in use of anesthetic gases.
3. Nonprovision of oxygen analyzers.

Cost of Volatile Agents

In order to present an economic argument, one must take into account the current costs of the items concerned. The cost of volatile agents in the UK in 1987 was of the order of £6.8 million. By volume, enflurane represented approximately half the total usage; isoflurane and halothane each accounted for about 25% of the total. By cost the picture is very different, isoflurane accounting for 54% of the total cost. In the UK today we pay about £32 per bottle for isoflurane. The manufacturer's recommended price is £33.50. The costing of volatile agents is complicated and not necessarily determined by the production cost. Figure 2 shows how external factors have influenced the cost of volatile agents. The cost of halothane has stayed steady at just over £5 per bottle. The three points marked on the figure indicate: (1) publication of a lead article in the *British Medical Journal* on the effect of halothane on the liver; (2) Anaquest cease supply of isoflurane in the UK, leaving a single supplier of this commodity; (3) Committe on Safety of Medicines' issued a warning on the use of halothane. These events have changed the pattern of usage of volatile agents.

In 1985, halothane accounted for 55% of the total volume used; in 1987 it had dropped to 25%. Use of isoflurane increased from 5 to 25% over the same period. So, if I had published this paper in 1986, a very different picture would have emerged. If an alternative agent were launched on the market tomorrow, for example, and the price of isoflurane cut in an attempt to retain its market share, the potential savings outlined later would not be achievable. In addition, what will be the effect on the cost of isoflurane when the patent expires in 1992? It may well be that some other manufacturer will decide to compete in this market, which could result in a reduction of the cost of isoflurane.

It is also important to note that the manufacturer's recommended price for isoflurane and enflurane has remained constant over the past five years at £33.50 and £33.35, respectively. Profits for the company who sell these products in the UK are controlled under the Phar-

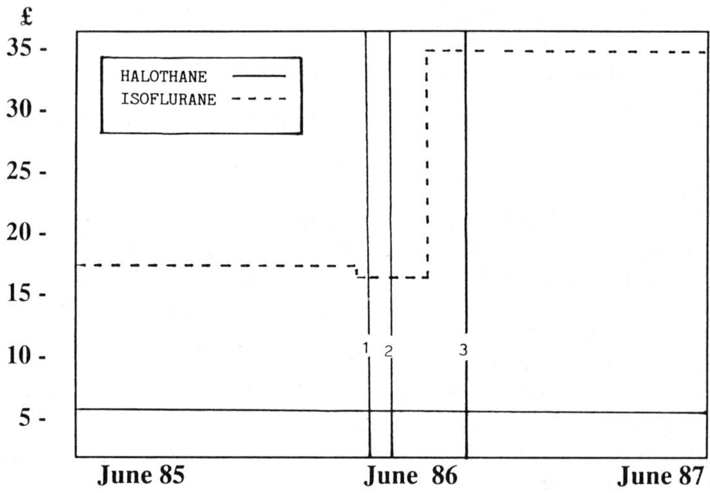

FIG. 2—*UK price fluctuation for volatile agents.*

maceutical Price Regulation Scheme (PPRS). The effect of this scheme and the effect on the possible outcome of any identifiable savings will be referred to later.

Thus the potential saving in volatile agents, accepting the earlier assumption, is therefore 40% of £6.8 million, i.e., £2.7 million (m).

Costs of Medical Gases

Again, costs for individual hospitals are not known, but the UK annual total for this commodity is in the region of £20 million for all medical purposes. Working on the assumption that 40% of the usage is in anesthesia, that represents about £8 million. With 40% reduction in usage, the potential saving is of the order of £3.2 million.

Costs of Oxygen Analyzers

As stated in the introduction, it is my intention to compare the cost of using an anesthetic machine with oxygen analyzer with those of the same anesthetic machine with gas monitoring systems. Thus if a gas monitor is used which has the capability of performing oxygen analysis, the cost of providing a separate analyzer is saved. An oxygen analyzer with alarm costs typically £400 with annual revenue costs of £150 (fuel cell, maintenance, and electricity). The estimated annual cost is therefore £230, representing a national expenditure of £0.9 million.

Summary of Savings

In summary, the savings amount to £2.7 m for the volatile agents, £3.2 m for medical gases, and £0.9 m for nonprovision of oxygen analyzers, making a total of £6.8 m.

Areas of Additional Expenditure

Expenditure associated with low-flow technique can be itemized as follows:

a. Provision of monitoring equipment, maintenance, and consumables costs.
b. Provision of CO_2 absorber and supply of soda lime.

Costs of Monitoring Equipment

There are a number of methods capable of determining the concentration of anesthetic agents and a number of types of commercially available equipment. I have chosen to consider laser Raman spectroscopy, piezoelectric detectors, and infrared absorption types. This selection covers a wide range of equipment costs. I have not included mass spectrometry because I was unable to obtain current costings and statistics and also because these are usually time-shared facilities and this presents additional problems when attempting to cost their use. The data necessary to do so on a national basis are not available.

The costs of the various techniques are given in Table 1. Typically, laser Raman equipment costs about £15 000, piezoelectric monitors are about £2000, and infrared instruments are about £6000. A fifth of these initial costs is taken as the annual cost. Added to this figure are the costs of 500 disposables (which is a very significant cost in some cases), calibration gases, servicing, and electricity. The latter is significant in the case of laser Raman, but less so for others. Because piezoelectric types cannot measure oxygen, the annual cost of an oxygen analyzer is added to this total in order to make it comparable with the others.

The total UK annual expenditure for these monitors is therefore £21.1 m, £16.9 m, and £2.9 m for laser Raman, infrared, and piezoelectric types, respectively.

It should be noted further that disposables for use with the monitors have been costed at the rate of one per session, i.e., 500 per annum. The UK agent for the Capnomac has indicated that gas sampling lines are disposable and priced at £7.10 each. They recommend that each sample line is used only once, but admit that in practice they have been used for up to nine months. Assuming four million operations are performed in the UK per annum, the cost of providing a new disposable for each case alone comes to £28.4 m, which outweighs the estimated savings by £21.6 m. I do, of course, recognize that the gas sample line will not be treated as a disposable item in practice, and I very much doubt that it will be replaced once per session, let alone once per case. If the running cost calculations are repeated, allowing £100 per annum for the provision of the disposable, a very different picture emerges. If the decision is taken not to replace these items in accordance with the manufacturer's instructions, the clinician must weigh the safety/litigation issues against the potential for saving money.

Costs of Soda Lime

The cost of providing soda lime is, contrary to the views expressed by some, significant. According to figures kindly provided by Dr. E. Schwanbom, for a typical adult (and assuming

TABLE 1—*Approximate annual costs for laser raman, piezoelectric, and infrared analyzers.*

Equipment Costs	Laser Raman, £15 000	Piezoelectric, £2000	Infrared, £6000
Annual cost	£3000	£400	£1200
Disposables (500 per annum)	£2500	N/A	£3500
Calibration gases	£250	£50	£50
Servicing	£100	£150	£70
Electricity	£178	neg.	£12
Oxygen analyzer	N/A	£230	N/A
Total	£6028	£830	£4832
National cost	£21.1 m	£2.9 m	£16.9 m
Limiting Cost of Disposables to £100 per Equipment			
National cost	£12.7 m	£2.9 m	£5.0 m

100% efficiency) 2 kg of soda lime will last for 1000 min. UK current costs are £7.84 for 4.5 kg, and assuming 2500 h operation per annum this gives an annual cost of £522. An absorber typically costs about £500, so the addition of this item to the anesthetic machine will add about £100 per annum to the total. Thus a grand total of £2.5 m is obtained as a national figure for expenditure.

Summary of Expenditure

In summary, the annual national cost for the provision of laser Raman equipment will be of the order of £21.1 m (£12.7 m with reduced disposable usage), £16.9 m for infrared instruments (£5.0 m), and £2.9 m for piezoelectric types. The cost of provision of soda lime is £2.5 m. The total national cost therefore is between £5.4 and £23.6 m depending on the type of monitoring equipment chosen.

Other Costs Not Considered

I ought to add that the manufacturer of the piezoelectric monitor, for example, states that if the sensor becomes contaminated it should be sterilized by ethylene oxide. If this is performed in a UK hospital, the cost of running a typical 4-ft^3 machine is approximately £120 per cycle. Of course one may be able to process several items together, in which case the cost of sterilization per item will be reduced. This and other incidental costs (e.g., provision of bacterial filters) are difficult to quantify and have therefore been excluded.

Potential Savings

Thus, theoretically, there is the potential for the UK to save about £1.4 million if the cheapest monitoring package is chosen. The other packages, even with reduced rates of disposable replacement, do not apparently generate savings.

There is a further question to be asked: Can the savings resulting from the use of the cheapest option actually be achieved?

Effect of PPRS

When discussing the costs of volatile agents I mentioned the Pharmaceutical Price Regulation Scheme. Briefly, it can be described as follows. Pharmaceutical companies who operate under the scheme are permitted to make an agreed overall profit dependent upon their total UK investment. Thus the profit on any particular item is decided by the company, providing the total profit for all products comes within the agreed amount. At the time of collecting the data for this paper (January 1989), both isofluorane (Forane) and enfluorane (Ethrane) were supplied under this scheme.

This permits the situation which occurred in 1986, where a doubling of the cost of enflurane and isoflurane was seen. As previously indicated, the UK isoflurane market was valued at £3.6 m in 1987. If low flow were to become the norm, the use of this agent would fall, and if there were no price adjustments, a £3.6 m business would be reduced to £2.2 m. Under these circumstances, the company that would probably still have the same manufacturing overheads (production plant, packaging lines, etc.) would presumably apply for a price increase. This would have a reasonable chance of success, i.e., overall the same profit could be made from the reduced turnover, which could result in an increase in cost of the volatile agent. Equally, and more probably, the company may choose not to increase the price of this commodity but to increase the price of one of its other lines. A similar argument can be made for the other agents.

Thus it may appear to NHS anesthetists that significant savings were being made, but the total NHS spend on pharmaceuticals would be unchanged. So from an overall view it is doubtful if the £2.7 m saving identified on volatile agents can really be achieved if everybody changes to low flow. It is interesting to note that the PPRS does not currently apply to medical gases so, in the absence of any price increase, the £3.7 m saving identified is unaffected.

Conclusions

It is my opinion that if the whole of the UK were to adopt low-flow techniques, costs would inevitably rise approximately by the amount required to install and run the monitoring equipment less any savings resulting from the reduction in use of medical gases. However, it is apparent that if a few hospitals change, then they are in the potential position of saving money if an appropriate analyzer is chosen.

It is clear that low-flow techniques and monitoring of anesthetic gases have advantages, some of which are difficult to quantify in economic terms, for example, reduction in theatre pollution, the movement of fewer cylinders, environmental issues, and increased patient safety. However, on the evidence provided I believe that it is inappropriate in the UK to justify the use of low-flow techniques by economic arguments alone.

The view expressed in this paper is that of the author and is not necessarily that held by the Department of Health.

Acknowledgments

Grateful thanks to all those who provided up-to-date information, particularly M. Halsey, J. Bushman, and E. Schwanbom.

Peter W. Thompson[1]

Conclusion and Summary for Standards Writing Purposes and Governmental Consideration

The origins of this meeting stemmed from International Organization for Standardization (ISO) Technical Committee 121 on Anaesthetic and Respiratory Equipment, Subcommittee 3 on Lung Ventilators and Related Equipment, who sought guidance as to whether it was appropriate or indeed necessary to propose as a new work item a standard for monitoring equipment for anesthetic vapor levels in the airways of patients or at the common gas outlet of the anesthesia machine.

The question we address in this publication is not one about the establishment of standards of anesthetic practice. It is not a question as to whether everyone should switch to low flow, or give it up, switch to opioids, or otherwise change their practice. It is whether ISO should write a new standard.

Readers of this publication will probably have been convinced that the technology is available, but that there are such wide variations in the performance of vaporizers that there might either be a cancelling out of the vaporizer error by an error in the monitor, or there might be a doubling of it, depending on whether the errors worked in the same or opposite directions.

Maybe we should be redesigning the vaporizer so that we can be absolutely sure of the concentration being delivered. I suggest this is not necessarily the whole answer because it does not take into account the behavior of vapors in low flow closed systems, which was, of course, examined by Mapleson [1], Galloon [2] and Mushin [3].

On balance, we should prepare a standard for anesthetic vapor monitors along the lines we have already for common gas outlet oxygen analyzers [4] and are nearing completion of for capnometry [5] and oximetry [6]. Moreover, a clear and completely testable declaration, verifiable by the test house, from the manufacturer about the performance of his equipment would be desirable both for anesthesia vapor monitors and for vaporizers.

References

[1] Mapleson, W. W., *British Journal of Anaesthesia*, Vol. 32, 1960, p. 298.
[2] Galloon, S., *British Journal of Anaesthesia*, Vol. 32, 1960, p. 310.
[3] Mushin, W. W. and Galloon, S., *British Journal of Anaesthesia*, Vol. 32, 1960, p. 324.
[4] International Organization for Standardization, "Particular Requirements for Safety of Oxygen Analyzers for Monitoring Patient Breathing Mixtures," ISO Standard No. 7767-1988, ISO, Geneva, 1988.
[5] International Organization for Standardization, "Capnometers for Use with Humans," ISO Standard No. 9918-1988, ISO, Geneva, 1988.
[6] International Organization for Standardization, "Pulse Oximeters for Medical Use—Safety Requirements," ISO Standard No. 9918-1988, ISO, Geneva, 1988.

[1]Department of Anaesthetics, University Hospital of Wales, Heath Park, Cardiff, CF4 4XW Wales, United Kingdom.